THE DISCIPLINE OF DIAGNOSIS

Cases and Visuals That Teach You How to Think

from The Clinical Problem Solvers

Rabih Geha, MD & Reza Manesh, MD

Edited by Tessa Kats-Rodgers

VOLUME 1

The Discipline of Diagnosis: Cases and Visuals That Teach You How to Think is a work of nonfiction. All patient identifying information has been modified to protect patient privacy.

This book is intended solely for educational purposes and does not constitute medical advice. It is not a substitute for professional medical judgment, diagnosis, or treatment. Clinical decisions should be made by qualified healthcare professionals based on the individual patient, clinical context, and current standards of care. While efforts have been made to ensure accuracy, the authors and publisher make no warranties regarding the completeness, timeliness, or reliability of the information presented. They expressly disclaim any liability for errors, omissions, or outcomes resulting from the use of this book.

Published in the United States by Clinical Problem Solvers

ISBN 978-1-7370983-3-1 Paperback

Cover and interior design by Asya Blue Design (asyablue.com)

For our learners, because of our patients

We owe a special thanks to Tessa for her editorial work on this book. Tessa graduated from high school this year (2026) and is the first high school student to subscribe to *RLRCPSolvers*. Aghajoon—Reza's grandfather—used to say that wisdom is not measured in years, and Tessa proves the point. Her instincts for language, rhythm, and clarity repeatedly made these pages better. Tessa, thank you for helping shape this book into something far stronger than what we started with.

Rabih Geha, MD, was born in Lebanon and spent much of his childhood in Pakistan before moving to the United States. There, he attended Boston College and later medical school at Brown University. He completed his residency in internal medicine and served as chief resident at UCSF. Rabih divides his clinical time between the emergency department and the inpatient teaching wards. He is particularly drawn to developing diagnostic schemas and building logical frameworks to approach clinical problems, a passion that traces back to his early interest in mathematics and the influence of his father.

Reza Manesh, MD, was born in Iran and grew up primarily in Pittsburgh. He graduated from the University of Pittsburgh School of Medicine and completed his internal medicine residency at UCSF. He works as a hospitalist, caring for patients alongside medical students and residents. Reza's passions include lifting heavy weights, eating at Chipotle, and studying in coffee shops. He credits his grandfather as his greatest inspiration. His ultimate goal is to share his excitement for and love of clinical problem-solving with others.

CONTENTS

FOREWORD

"You have to hear this."

Those were the words that started it all.

We had just settled onto kitchen stools to catch up after Austin returned from *The Society of Hospital Medicine Conference* in 2019. Once we started, we couldn't stop talking about what he had witnessed: a physician standing before a room of clinicians—many far more experienced—working through a clinical case in real time. No prior knowledge. No cues. Just his mind, his method, and a willingness to think out loud.

It wasn't a performance; it was a masterclass. Rather than racing toward a diagnosis, the physician was revealing how one was made: the pivots, the probabilities, and the reasoning behind every question. It was clinical reasoning, not as a conclusion, but as a living process.

That physician? Rabih Geha.

A few weeks later, we found *The Clinical Problem Solvers* podcast and couldn't stop listening. At the time, we were second-year internal medicine residents living together, and the podcast quickly became a ritual. With each new piece of information, we would pause, turn toward each other, and work through the case ourselves—testing hypotheses, naming uncertainties, and committing to a line of reasoning before pressing play again.

Those weren't just enjoyable evenings. They were deliberate practice—reps that sharpened how we thought, how we taught, and how we navigated uncertainty. More than that, they reintroduced something easy to lose in training: the sense that medicine, even at its most complex, could still be deeply engaging—even fun.

Months later, Reza and Rabih discussed a case together at *The Society to Improve Diagnosis in Medicine Conference* with Alec there to bear witness. We found ourselves back in the kitchen afterward, reflecting once again.

Seeing their work live revealed something that even the best podcast episode could not fully capture. There was clinical excellence, of course, but also something more enduring: composure under pressure, humility in the face of uncertainty, and a generosity of spirit that made their expertise feel accessible rather than intimidating. And threaded through it all was the beauty and power of partnership. A genuine brotherhood.

As identical twins, we recognized that bond immediately. The innate closeness. The banter you can only get away with when trust and love are deeply embedded. The way one person's passion ignites the other.

In the years since, we've watched Reza and Rabih grow, not only as clinicians and educators but also as partners in a shared intellectual project. Each has absorbed something of the other's strengths, and their commitment to reflection, humility, and improvement has only deepened. Just as importantly, they have chosen to extend that growth to an eager community—one that is as committed to continuous learning as they are.

That initiative began as a podcast but has since grown into something much larger. *The Clinical Problem Solvers* is now a global educational community dedicated to improving how clinicians think, grounded in a simple but powerful idea: that excellent clinical reasoning should not be confined by geography, institutional affiliation, or access to elite training environments.

This commitment is not abstract; it reflects lived experience. Before training together, Reza and Rabih had each seen how the quality of clinical reasoning—and the opportunity to develop it—could vary widely. They recognized that the gap was not one of talent, but of access. Through freely available teaching, widely shared diagnostic schemas, and a growing international network of learners, they have worked to narrow that gap. *The Clinical Problem Solvers Academy*—of which we remain proud members—is one expression of that effort. It is a model of what can happen when high standards and open access are pursued together.

This book represents the fullest realization of their vision.

It is, at once, a masterwork of clinical reasoning and a genuine pleasure to read. Reza and Rabih bring their whole selves to it: the banter, the vulnerability, and the moments of real tension when the stakes are someone's loved one—maybe even their own.

You'll encounter complex cases rendered with the clarity of great teaching, but you'll experience them like a compelling novel: drawn in, unsettled, surprised. You'll laugh. You'll feel the weight of what it means to take care of people at their most vulnerable. And along the way, you'll absorb something that no exam can test—an orientation toward medicine that is rigorous, humble, and deeply human. You will also come to understand that no matter where you're starting from, being your authentic self, staying diligent in your commitment to learning, and growing from your mistakes are all you need to join them on the road to excellence.

We imagine that, as you read this book, you will find yourself thinking a little differently—more deliberate in your reasoning, more comfortable with uncertainty, and perhaps even more connected to the part of medicine that first drew you to it.

We are better clinicians and better people because of Rabih and Reza. We suspect you will be too.

Alec & Austin Rezigh

INTRODUCTION

WHY THIS IS NOT A TEXTBOOK

We didn't write this book to teach you all of medicine.

There are already shelves full of excellent textbooks that do that better than we ever could. This book exists for a different reason: to share how we learned medicine, how we continue to learn medicine, and why we believe that approach can make you better, regardless of your specialty, training level, or where you practice.

What we found early on is that the difference between clarity and confusion rarely comes down to how much you know. It often results from what you do when the answer isn't obvious. Do you rush to closure? Or do you generate possibilities, test them against reality, and change course when the facts refuse to cooperate?

We are Rabih and Reza. We trained together in internal medicine at UCSF, surrounded by mentors who showed us something powerful early on. We learned that diagnosis is not just a destination. It is a discipline of thought. A way of seeing patients more clearly, asking better questions, and staying engaged long after each encounter ends.

Before procedures or treatments enter the picture, our most consequential tool is how we think. Diagnosis shapes prognosis and guides treatment. It answers the three questions patients care about most: What do I have? What can be done about it? What does this mean for me long term? In an era of rapid technological change, artificial intelligence (AI) tools like OpenEvidence have become a prevalent part of that diagnostic process. While they put vast medical knowledge within immediate reach, they serve to supplement, not replace the disciplined reasoning, unwavering empathy, and insatiable curiosity of a well-trained clinician.

For Rabih, that curiosity is personal. His father's diagnosis of Parkinson's disease was delayed by nearly a decade. Constipation dismissed. Sleep disrupted but ignored. Tremors explained away. And watching symptoms accumulate without clarity left a lasting imprint. It shaped a lifelong commitment to understanding how and why diagnoses are missed, delayed, or misunderstood, so others do not have to endure what his father did.

For Reza, the spark came from a different place. He realized that when he truly understood why something was happening, he could both teach it more effectively and treat patients more thoughtfully. Reflecting on his own journey, he came to see that deep understanding was essential, not just for mastering information, but for connecting it meaningfully to patient care. Clinical reasoning is what makes that connection possible. It bridges what we know, what we say, and how patients actually experience their care. Without it, knowledge fragments, communication falters, and even well-intentioned treatment can miss the mark.

Though our experiences differed, they led us to the same question: How do smart, caring clinicians miss what matters most?

Over the past decade, we have dedicated ourselves to learning diagnostic reasoning the way most clinicians authentically encounter medicine: through real cases. Not idealized vignettes. Not board-style one-liners. Real patients, real uncertainty, real cognitive missteps. Each case led us to pause, reflect, draw figures, revisit assumptions, and refine our thinking. Then repeat. Again and again.

The figures you will see throughout this book are not perfect. We kept them that way on purpose. Imperfect. Human. Thought in motion. They began as our Picasso: an iPad, Evernote, a stylus, and many early mornings with coffee while Rabih's dog, Naar, barked to play with his favorite orange-red ball and Reza's cats, Geno and Sid, meowed for Greenies. We hope you engage with them the same way we do—not as polished conclusions, but as thinking tools you can redraw, adapt, and make your own.

Some readers will move quickly through the cases and glance at the figures as they go. Others will pause, study them, and flip to the appendix for a fuller explanation. We designed it this way on purpose. However you read, we hope the diagnostic maps sharpen your thinking.

For readers who want to go deeper, the appendix becomes a master class in the figures themselves. There, we walk through each diagram in detail, explaining how every element on the page connects to physiology, base rates, and the clinical priorities that shape real decisions, including recognizing dangerous diagnoses that cannot be missed. The goal is not just to decode the figures but to show how they tell a coherent story. A single visual framework can organize complexity and make the reasoning behind a concept visible.

Added together, we've likely spent more than 40,000 combined hours thinking about cases, teaching them, breaking them apart, and putting them back together again.

This book is our attempt to share what came out of that process.

WHAT THIS BOOK IS (AND ISN'T)

This is not a book organized by organ system. It is not a list of diseases you must memorize. And it is definitely not a promise that you'll know everything when you're done. Instead, this book follows 21 real cases, most drawn from our *RLRCPSolvers* podcast series, that challenged us, unsettled us, and forced us to revise our thinking. Most cases unfold from our shared point of view, with moments where the lens narrows to Rabih, to Reza, or moves fluidly between us as the reasoning evolves.

The cases are authentic. The uncertainty is authentic. The identifying details are not. We make acknowledging uncertainty a core aspect of this book rather than pretending it does not exist.

Each chapter begins where medicine actually begins: with an incomplete story. As the cases unfold, so does our reasoning, including branch points, moments of hesitancy, diagnostic pivots, and the quiet skills that rarely make it into textbooks.

Throughout the book, you will see moments labeled "**Pause and Reflect.**" These are not rhetorical questions. They are invitations to stop and decide what you would do next before we illuminate our reasoning.

Yes, diagnoses matter.

But just as often, the deeper learning is about how we think, how we care, and how we grow. Ultimately, we must consider the following:

- How to recognize when a pattern is misleading and how to slow down when your brain wants to sprint
- How to continue caring even when you cannot offer a clear diagnosis or effective treatment
- How to forgive yourself as you learn, knowing you are a work in progress and will make mistakes

We didn't choose these cases because of their final diagnoses. We chose them because the reasoning inside them matters.

THE REAL GOAL

Our hope is not that you finish this book knowing more facts but that you finish it thinking differently about the next patient you see. If this book succeeds, it will inspire you to pause after your own cases, to ask what surprised you, what you missed, and what you might alter in your future actions. That habit—more than any single diagnosis—is how experience slowly turns into growth and expertise.

Above all, this book is an invitation into our journey of clinical reasoning. We're grateful you're here for it.

Let's get started.

1

It was 10 p.m. Pacific. Reza was half asleep, hovering in that thin space between dream and pager-brain, when his phone lit up on the nightstand. He reached for it without thinking.

"Hey, can I ask you a question?"

It was 1 a.m. where she was on the East Coast. Reza stared at the screen for a moment, reading it twice as his mind flickered on.

He called. No answer.

He FaceTimed. Her face filled the screen, dimly lit by a small bedside lamp. She was sitting upright against the headboard.

She looked tired. Not just sleepy, but worn down. "Hey," she said quietly. "Can you hear me? I'm trying not to wake Lenny." Lenny was her 15-pound shih tzu who vaguely resembled a lentil.

The words, even in her quiet tone, landed wrong. Her voice sounded dulled, not hoarse or breathy but thick and nasal. She tried to smile, likely catching the shift in Reza's expression. He reached over and turned on the light beside his bed.

"Say that again."

"Which part?" she asked.

He needed to hear more. Volume, resonance, the way air moved. "Just say a full sentence."

She eyed him warily but complied. "I'm fine. It just really hurts."

The words came out muffled, like she was speaking through a barrier.

"Are you drooling?"

A small shake of her head. "No."

"Can you swallow?"

She paused, and Reza watched her do it deliberately, the effort visible in her neck. "Yes. It hurts."

"Any trouble breathing?"

She inhaled slowly before answering, almost as if she were checking it for the first time. "No." Then, more quietly: "Am I okay?"

Before giving advice, his shoulders tightened. He sat up, elbows knocking lightly against the bed frame.

He was her brother, older by ten years. For as long as he could remember, he'd felt the need to look out for her. To protect her.

But he was also a doctor. He had seen how quickly anatomy could turn. A small space swelling shut. A voice changing. Air moving a little slower with each breath.

Reza's mind instinctively drifted to Rabih, whose advice he often leaned on when a case felt off. But right now, it was just him and his sister, talking through a screen.

"Hold on," he said. "Let's go back. How did it start?"

"A sore throat, ten-ish days ago," she replied. "It felt like someone was stabbing me."

She had just returned from another stretch of travel. Boston. London. Tokyo. Always moving, city to city, until finally coming home.

Pause and Reflect

What principle helps you distinguish viral from bacterial pharyngitis?

The key was pattern recognition. Viral illness tended to be diffuse—cough, congestion, myalgias, conjunctivitis, hoarseness—inflammation spreading across systems rather than staying in one place.

Bacterial pharyngitis, by contrast, tended to localize. The pain centered in the throat, often abrupt, without widespread upper respiratory symptoms.

Before moving forward, it helps to visualize how the diagnostic branches separate.

Figure 1.1

Diagnostic Approach to Pharyngitis

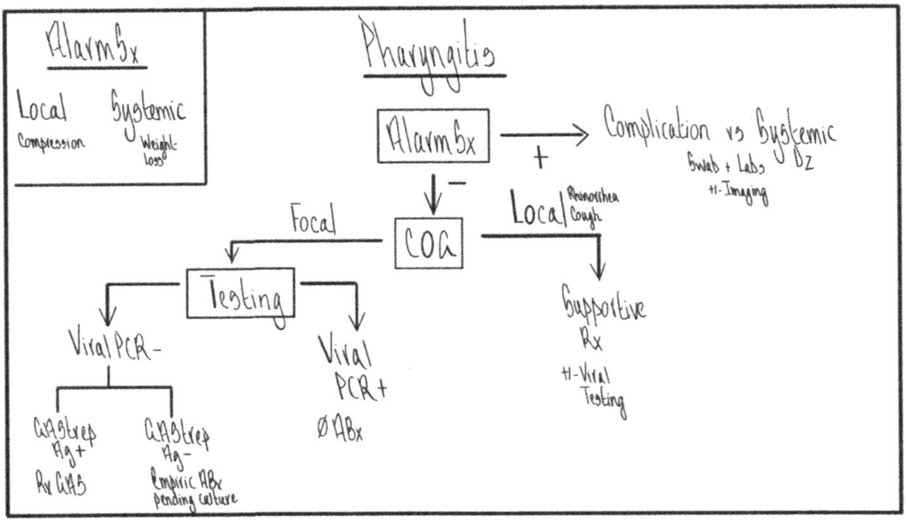

This map helps us decide whether an illness is a focal throat-centered syndrome, which raises concern for bacterial pharyngitis, or part of a broader viral process.

"Any cough?"

She shook her head.

"Congestion? Runny nose? Muscle aches?"

She looked at him the way she always did when he slipped into doctor mode. A little amused, a little tired. "No. Just my throat."

That answer was enough to change the frame. The diffuse signature of a viral illness wasn't there.

"The first place I went was urgent care."

Rapid strep testing was negative. Influenza, RSV, and COVID testing were also negative. The illness was attributed to viral pharyngitis, and a methylprednisolone dose pack was prescribed for the pain.

But bacterial pharyngitis wasn't limited to *Group A Strep*. It included organisms a rapid test wouldn't catch: non–group A streptococci, *Fusobacterium* in younger adults, and other anaerobes hiding in tonsillar crypts.

"I felt amazing the next day."

Steroids eased inflammation, no doubt. But it was entirely plausible that the methylprednisolone could make her feel better while an infection continued to evolve underneath. Relief was persuasive. It could rewrite the story. She completed the six-day taper, with the steroid course stopping on day seven. The pain returned less than a day later, stronger than before. She told him she sat through class barely able to focus, counting down to her next ibuprofen, every swallow landing like shards of glass.

She saw primary care the afternoon before they FaceTimed. Vital signs were normal. Her throat was erythematous. The white blood cell count was 14,000.

"Probably steroids," the primary care doctor said, referring to the leukocytosis.

Steroids could cause leukocytosis through demargination, usually appearing early and declining with cessation. A white count of 14,000 at the tail end of a taper could fit that explanation.

It would have been easy to leave it there. To protect the original frame and bend new information to fit it.

Then his sister spoke again. "It's only on one side."

That broke the pattern.

He asked her to open her mouth and angle the camera with the flashlight on. The right side looked fuller.

She now had a fever of 100.6°F despite alternating acetaminophen and ibuprofen. This was no longer a nuisance syndrome. Her voice thickened. The right soft palate bulged toward midline. Anatomy was claiming space.

Peritonsillar abscess until proven otherwise.

At this point, the question shifts from diagnosis to anatomy and spread.

Figure 1.2

Suppurative Complications of Pharyngitis

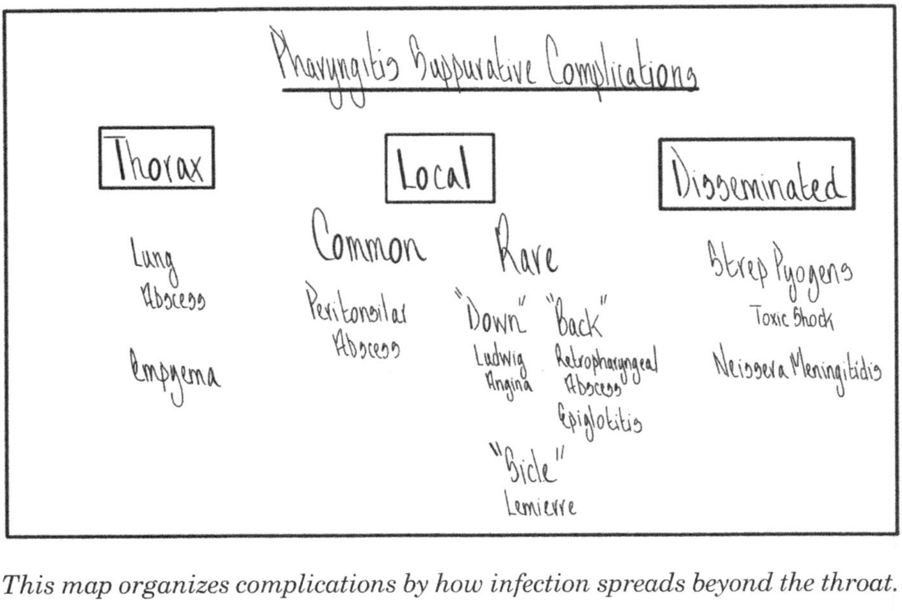

This map organizes complications by how infection spreads beyond the throat.

She had an ENT appointment scheduled for the next afternoon. Twelve hours away.

Going to the emergency department at 1 a.m. meant long waits, tests, consults, and exhaustion before treatment even began. Nevertheless, she asked, voice wavering, "Should I go?"

The screen went quiet, and Reza could see her waiting. He had to decide.

Pause and Reflect

Would you send her to the ED?

Although most peritonsillar abscesses were treated outside the hospital, suspicion for upper airway compromise changed the threshold.

Reza told her to go. Not because he was certain she would obstruct, but because he could not safely rule it out through a screen. She went.

After they hung up, he turned off his nightstand light and walked into the living room. The apartment was quiet; it felt strangely like being on an overnight shift—awake, alert, and waiting for updates. Fortunately, his cat Sidney kept him company, lying on his chest and purring as if he knew his owner was distressed.

There were delays. His sister texted updates from the triage bay. Then from room 7.

Eventually, the answer came, not as reassurance but as data. A CT with contrast revealed a three-by-three-centimeter peritonsillar abscess. ENT was subsequently consulted.

Then there was more waiting. Every time Reza's phone vibrated, he grabbed it instantly. Once, as he began to drift off, he thought he felt the phone buzz, only to realize it was Sid purring beside him. Around 4 a.m. the messages stopped for a while. Eventually, he gave in and slept.

Reza woke to his phone vibrating against his chest. For a moment he just stared at the screen, his palms damp, hoping the message would say what he needed it to say. It did. At 7 a.m., her time, they drained the abscess.

Relief, this time, came with specifics. Pus returned. Cultures later grew *Group A Strep*. A few days after drainage, she felt better. Soft diet, voice restored, pain gone.

Later that day, she sent Reza a photo of a milkshake with Lenny hovering beside it, ready to strike. "First thing I could swallow," she wrote. Only then did he relax, indulging in a Chipotle bowl with extra sour cream, his body craving something greasy after a night deprived of quality sleep.

Someone later suggested, after a recounting of the story, that she could have waited for the clinic appointment. Maybe.

But maybe was not a strategy in a narrow space.

Recap

- When pharyngitis presents without a cough or additional upper respiratory symptoms, bacterial causes should move higher on the differential, and *Group A Strep* is not the only causative organism.
- Steroids can dramatically improve symptoms but may mask progression and increase the risk of suppurative complications.
- When upper airway compromise is possible, accept a few overcalls; obstruction is not a complication diagnosed retrospectively.

2

They were in the middle of an arthrocentesis. Rabih held the syringe steady, aspirating fluid from a swollen knee that had been bothering their patient for days. The plunger resisted, then gave with a soft release, cloudy fluid slipping into the syringe. They were debating crystals versus infection when the nurse appeared at the curtain.

"Sorry to interrupt. One of you needs to come. Room 14."

There was an odd tone in her voice, not panic, but just tight enough to notice.

The patient caught their debate as Reza stepped out. He turned toward Rabih with a tired shake of his head.

"Doc," he said, "of course it's gout."

Room 14 held an older man with diabetes and chronic venous stasis. His left leg was red and tense, the erythema spreading from mid-ankle toward the knee in uneven borders. His temperature was 100.7°F. Blood pressure stable. Heart rate normal.

Familiar territory. Red. Warm. Tender. Fever.

Reza examined the leg carefully, pressing gently against the skin. The erythema was irregular but clear. Warmth radiated through his gloves into his fingertips, while the tenderness drew a grimace around the patient's eyes.

"That's pretty sore, huh?" Reza asked.

"Yeah," the patient exhaled.

Classic cellulitis. The kind diagnosed on the walk in. Reza checked the right leg. Chronic stasis changes. No warmth. No redness. No tenderness.

"We'll start antibiotics, keep your leg elevated, and run some labs," Reza explained.

His hand reached for the doorknob. The patient shifted hesitantly.

"Oh, and doc?"

Reza turned back.

"My other leg is starting to feel like this one did yesterday. Not red yet. But the same deep ache."

Reza paused, his hand still on the door handle. The hallway noise drifted in behind him. The exam had been normal. But he stayed at the door a second longer, listening to the uncertainty in the man's voice.

"Alright," he replied. "We'll keep monitoring it."

He stepped out, but the comment followed him down the hallway—unacted upon but not forgotten.

Back in the other room, Rabih was sealing the arthrocentesis sample with deliberate care.

"Fluid looked inflammatory. We'll see if it's crystals or infection."

Reza nodded. "Room 14 is straightforward. Left leg cellulitis. Fever. Diabetes."

"Good," Rabih answered. "Bread and butter."

Reza hesitated. "But as I was leaving, he said the right leg is starting to feel the same way. No redness yet; just a deep ache."

Rabih leaned back slightly. "That's unusual," he said. "Cellulitis is usually unilateral. It rarely affects both legs at once."

Reza nodded. "Unless there's skin breakdown on both legs creating a vulnerability to infection, but there's no evidence of that."

They treated the comment as provisional data. Not diagnostic, but directional enough to remember. One leg was objectively abnormal; the other was not. A left-dominant process with fever. Base rate still favored cellulitis. They started antibiotics, elevated the leg, marked the borders, and sent labs. Blood cultures were drawn, more out of hospital reflex than necessity, and the patient was admitted for social reasons. Still, the memory persisted—that brief pause at the door before the story felt complete.

Pause and Reflect

What are cellulitis mimics?

They ran the usual decoys. DVT. Stasis dermatitis. Gout. The problem was the fever and the heat. Those pushed infection back to the top, with necrotizing infection sitting off to the side like a shark fin: unlikely but never ignorable.

When one leg is red and swollen, we must organize the problem before we label it.

Figure 2.1

Approach to unilateral leg erythema and swelling

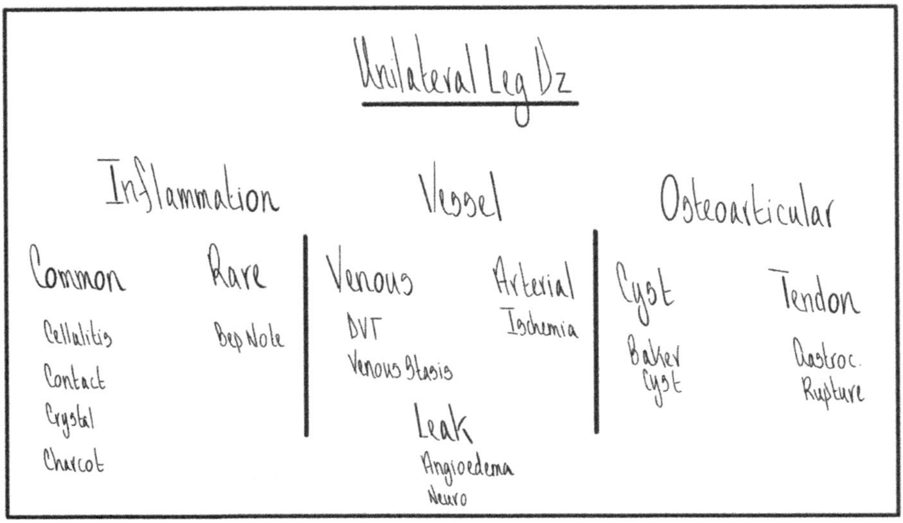

Unilateral leg findings can arise from inflammation, vascular issues, or osteoarticular pathology.

Day 1 labs: white count 11, CRP 30. Reasonable.

Day 2 brought an accidentally repeated CRP of 300. Reza stared at the number, his earlier uncertainty resurfacing.

“That’s not how simple cellulitis behaves.”

The number mattered, but so did its direction. A rising inflammatory marker, even without dramatic clinical change, suggested the story was still evolving. The left leg looked much the same.

Then the patient asserted, “My right leg feels worse now.”

They examined it again, finding a faint pink hue above the ankle, easy to miss unless you were looking for it.

Reza entered the workroom, momentum returning. “It’s declaring itself.”

The case was no longer unilateral cellulitis.

Rabih looked at him, spinning around in his chair. “Now it’s sequential.”

Pause and Reflect

What is your next diagnostic move?

They widened their concern to the most dangerous miss, not because it explained the case yet, but because it could not be ignored. They checked the sodium and ordered imaging.

CT scan: *no necrotizing fasciitis. Soft tissue stranding consistent with cellulitis.*

Microbiology was called. Two out of two blood cultures returned with gram-negative rods.

Reza walked to Rabih’s desk, his mind whirring.

“Not staph. Not strep.”

Rabih raised an eyebrow. “That doesn’t fit typical cellulitis.” He thought aloud, slowing the frame, “Outside bugs are usually gram-positive. Gram-negatives make you think about an inside source.”

Reza went back into the patient’s room. Before he could ask about pets, his phone buzzed. A text from Rabih: “Gram-negative rod finalized.

Think cats."

When skin turns red, we reflexively think about strep and staph. But once the blood cultures shift the frame, the map changes.

Figure 2.2

Cellulitis and gram-negative rods

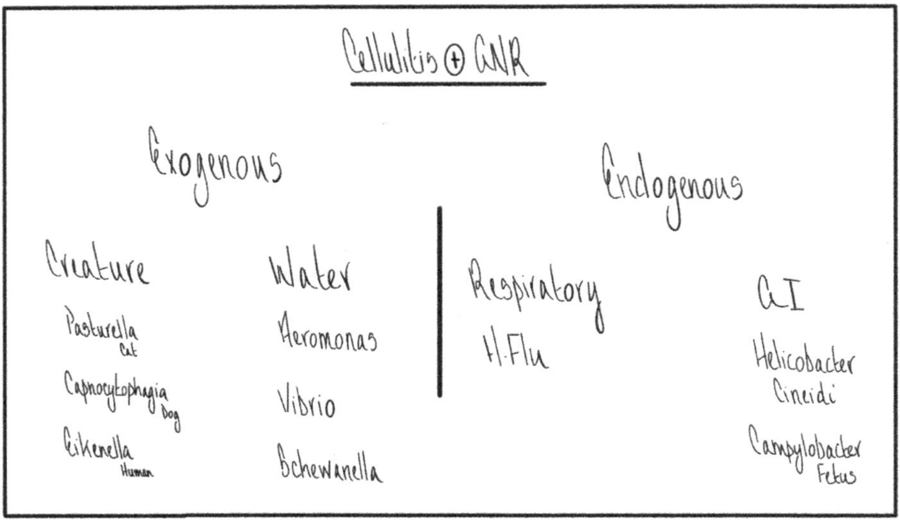

Typical cellulitis is caused by gram-positive skin bacteria, but gram-negative organisms suggest an unusual exposure or an endogenous source of infection.

"Any cats?"

"Four," the patient answered.

"Bites?"

"No."

"Scratches?"

"Not that I remember."

"Licks?"

"Certainly."

Reza smiled and retrieved his phone from his pocket. "I have two orange cats. Sid and Geno." He shook his head. "Absolute chaos."

He scrolled through his photos until he found a good one. Geno sprawled across a keyboard; Sidney wedged behind a monitor. "Geno climbs onto my pillow at two in the morning and scratches it until I give him Greenies. Sid waits until three and paws my face until I pet him." He turned his phone toward the patient. "I haven't slept through the night since 2013."

The patient laughed. "Mine sleep on my legs every night."

For a moment they traded pictures, orange fur glowing under bedside lamps. The pathophysiology landed differently when it arrived wrapped in something familiar.

Now the sequence made sense. Cat scratch, bite, or lick. Unilateral cellulitis. Bacteremia. Hematogenous seeding. Sequential skin involvement.

The right leg hadn't been noise. It had been the earliest clue, spoken quietly before the exam ever changed.

Pause and Reflect

Name the bug.

Pasteurella multocida.

The first story fit beautifully: unilateral cellulitis in a diabetic patient. When the CRP rose, they could have simply called it worse cellulitis, but that would have been inconsistent with the exam, which looked largely unchanged. Instead, a single comment at the doorknob kept pulling them back toward uncertainty.

The patient improved on ceftriaxone and transitioned to amoxicillin-clavulanate. Before discharge, they talked again about the cats. The patient smiled and made it clear he was not changing a thing.

As they left the ED that night, Rabih glanced over at Reza. "Good catch earlier."

Reza shook his head. "He caught it. We just listened."

Later that night, the arthrocentesis results returned: gout. Rabih texted, *"Sometimes the patient already knows the ending. We just spend the chapter catching up."*

Recap

- Nearly a third of cellulitis diagnoses are mimics such as stasis dermatitis, DVT, or gout.
- Bilateral cellulitis is exceptionally rare. When erythema is bilateral, think shared exposure or, far less commonly, hematogenous seeding from select organisms such as *Vibrio vulnificus*.
- When a patient raises a concern that does not fit the first story, resist immediately dismissing it. It may be unrelated, but it also might be the key to the diagnosis.

3

It was just past midnight in the emergency department, the hour when decisions felt heavier because fewer people were awake. The workroom was nearly empty, with just two people inside. A half-finished cup of coffee sat between Rabih and Reza, cooling beside an open chart. The shift had settled into that uneasy quiet, where you could almost fall for the illusion of calm.

Rabih scrolled through labs from earlier in the evening, slowing over numbers the way he always did when he sensed a pattern forming.

Reza dictated a note into the microphone, finishing documentation on a patient he had just treated for hypertension.

"Hypertension."

Nothing.

He tried again. "Hypertension."

The screen confidently offered: *Hyperthyroidism.*

Rabih didn't look up. "Careful. You're about one repetition away from an endocrine consult."

Reza leaned closer to the microphone. "Hy-per-ten-sion."

The cursor blinked. Then: *Hyper tension.*

He sat back. Then forward again. "Hypertension."

Still wrong.

"Hypertension!"

Finally, the word appeared correctly.

Reza stared at the screen for a beat. "Unbelievable."

Then Rabih's phone vibrated against the desk. He glanced at the screen and straightened slightly. "It's one of my primary care patients."

He answered and put the call on speaker, letting the caller know he was doing so, so his colleague could listen in and help. She agreed.

It was the patient's wife speaking. Her voice was steady at first, but the strain surfaced quickly. She had gone into the bathroom after her husband and found the toilet bowl bright red, blood on the floor beside it.

"He feels fine. But I saw blood."

The patient was seventy-two with advanced dementia. No fever. No flank pain. No abdominal pain. No urinary complaints. He insisted nothing hurt, but she knew he could not reliably tell her when something was wrong.

Pause and Reflect

What is the most important thing to clarify?

Before narrowing the problem, it helps to step back and categorize how bleeding behaves.

Figure 3.1

Hemorrhage Overview: Open vs Closed Spaces

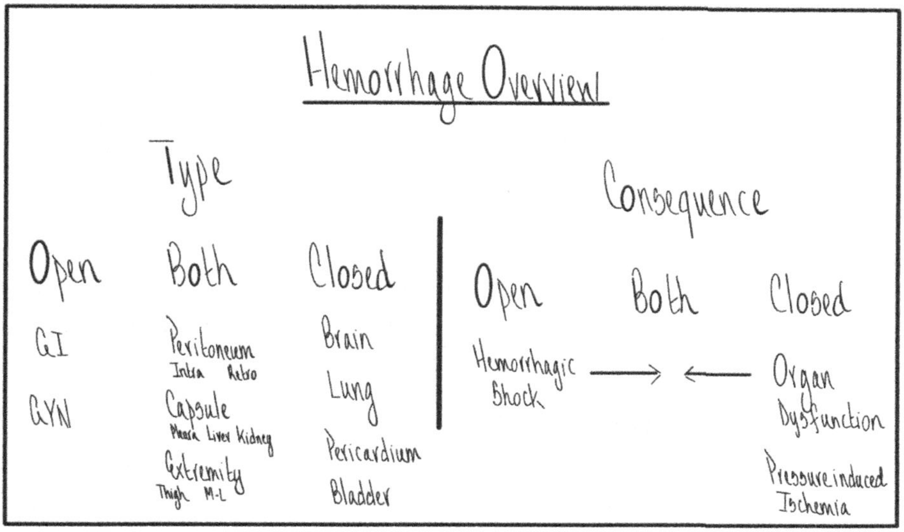

The location of bleeding determines the dominant threat: volume loss in open systems or pressure in closed compartments.

Reza felt the pull toward reassurance. The instinct to calm fear before the facts came into focus.

Rabih slowed the moment down. "First we orient," he said, glancing at Reza. "Help me localize this."

Bleeding required orientation before explanation. The first question was not why. It was where. Blood in a toilet bowl pulled your brain toward GI pathology. But appearances were often deceiving. The source could be urinary, rectal, cutaneous, or, when relevant, gynecologic.

Rabih kept his tone gentle. "Can you check his underwear and around his penis?"

There was a pause on the line. They heard the phone being set down, the small sounds of movement on the other end. When she returned, her breath was shaky.

"There's blood at the tip," she murmured. "And small clots."

Reza felt the frame click into place. Urinary source.

Rabih rubbed his chin. "Okay. That helps a lot."

If a urinalysis were available, microscopy would confirm the source; the dipstick detected heme, not intact red blood cells. But none of that existed tonight. They were sitting inside an emergency department while the problem unfolded miles away. No scanner. No catheter. Just questions.

Rabih listened closely. Clots mattered. They implied focal bleeding, something beyond the glomerulus. Reza was already thinking the same thing: a plumbing problem until proven otherwise.

The immediate danger was obstruction. Clots could block the outlet. Pressure could rise. The bladder could stop emptying. At that moment, the diagnosis was secondary information. First came the essential question: was the bladder still functioning?

Pause and Reflect

What would you ask his wife to decide whether he needs to go to the emergency department?

Reza moved into checklist mode. "Is he having lower belly pain? Any pressure like he needs to pee but can't? Is he passing urine?"

They listened. None were present. No pain. No retention. No instability.

Rabih exhaled slowly. "Most hematuria doesn't require the ED tonight."

They recommended liberal oral fluids and scheduled voiding every two to three hours while awake. Simple steps to maintain flow and prevent clots from accumulating.

Restraint, not inaction.

Only once safe bladder function was established did they step back to classify the bleeding. Clots supported a nonglomerular source.

Rabih worked through the framework aloud. Infection, stones, trauma, malignancy.

With obstruction ruled out, the next step is to localize where blood is entering the urinary tract.

Figure 3.2

Hematuria: An Anatomic Approach

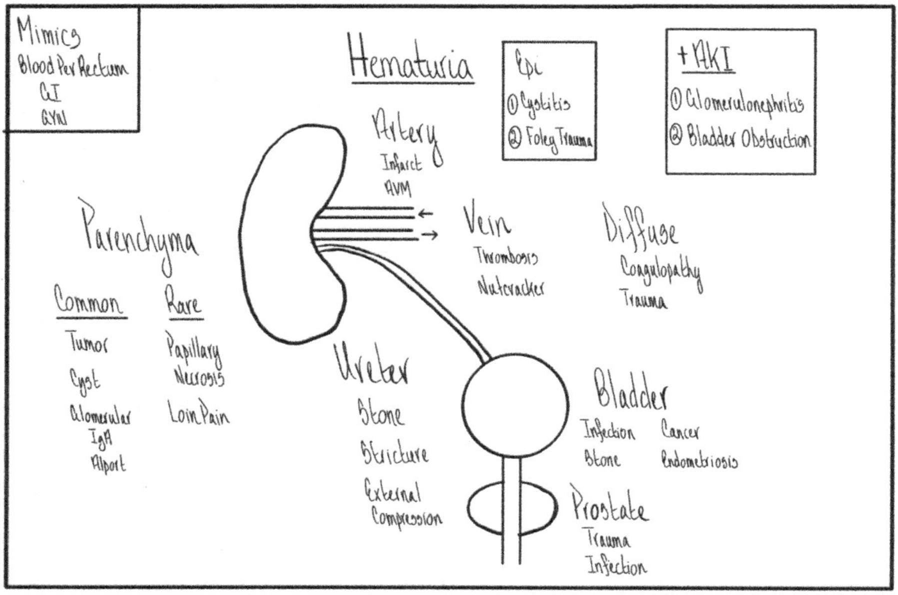

Identifying where blood is entering the urinary tract focuses the differential and directs evaluation.

The wife went quiet for a moment. When she spoke again, something had shifted in her tone. "Is this cancer?"

"It's something we need to evaluate," Rabih answered. "But it's not the most common cause."

Reza added, "Many episodes like this are temporary. We still investigate fully, but it doesn't automatically mean cancer."

The silence that followed felt different from the earlier instance. Not panicked. Processing.

Then: "So we don't go to the hospital tonight?"

"Not unless he stops urinating, develops pain, or seems uncomfortable," Reza replied. "You'd know. Trust yourself."

"Okay." Her voice had steadied, and she repeated, like self-reassurance, "Okay."

Rabih ended the call and set the phone down on the desk. Their monitors were still on in the background, flickering. Reza reached for his coffee, found it cold, and set it down again. Neither of them rushed to say anything.

Then Rabih clicked into the chart, and they reviewed the next steps for the patient. Upper tract imaging with CT urogram. Lower tract evaluation with cystoscopy. Different tools for different anatomy.

The patient's next void was clear. He remained asymptomatic.

Still, gross hematuria in older adults required full evaluation. Transient bleeding was not reassurance.

The workup continued in an outpatient setting. CT urogram negative. Cystoscopy negative. No malignancy. It ended with no clear cause: nonglomerular hematuria, unexplained but reassuringly benign.

What stayed with them was not the diagnosis itself, but how easily fear could have pushed everyone toward unnecessary escalation. Sometimes the quiet win in medicine was not what you found but what you avoided doing too soon.

Recap

- When blood appears, the first task is orientation, not diagnosis. Identifying where bleeding originates and whether it is trapped or escaping prevents missed danger and unnecessary escalation.
- Gross hematuria is a plumbing problem until proven otherwise. The key branch point is whether obstruction is developing.
- Clinical reasoning does not stop when the patient is at home. Clear instructions, physiologic thinking, and restraint can protect patients just as effectively as aggressive escalation.

4

Rabih and Reza sat in their usual seats in the emergency department, monitors angled toward each other. Morning light cut across the workstation as the tracking board refreshed, a new name appearing at the top with an uncommon chief concern.

"Rectal pain," Reza read aloud.

Rabih swiveled slightly in his chair. "That tends to localize itself."

Rectal pain was different from abdominal pain. When someone said, "my stomach hurts," the differential widened quickly. When someone said, "my rectum hurts," anatomy narrowed the field before they could ask another question. The patient had already localized the problem for them; their task was now to decide whether the pain truly behaved like a local process.

A few minutes later, in the exam room, the patient lowered himself toward the chair and paused halfway, his jaw tightening. He shifted his weight, exhaled through his nose, and finally settled onto one hip.

"Doc, it hurts so bad I can't sit."

He hesitated, then added quietly, almost apologetically, "It's inside. In my rectum. It's been a week."

After a moment, he went on, "It's worst when I try to go."

The patient was thirty-two years old. The pain was constant, about a seven out of ten, rising to unbearable levels during bowel movements. No fevers, no chills. No systemic symptoms he could name. The vitals were normal. The abdominal exam was benign.

Reza caught Rabih's eye for a split second. Well appearing did not mean comfortable.

They examined the anus. Nothing. No fissure, no hemorrhoid, no wart, no obvious lesion. That was usually where doctors stopped.

Before going further, it helps to visualize the branching anatomy of anorectal pain.

Figure 4.1

Anorectal Pain: An Exam-Driven Framework

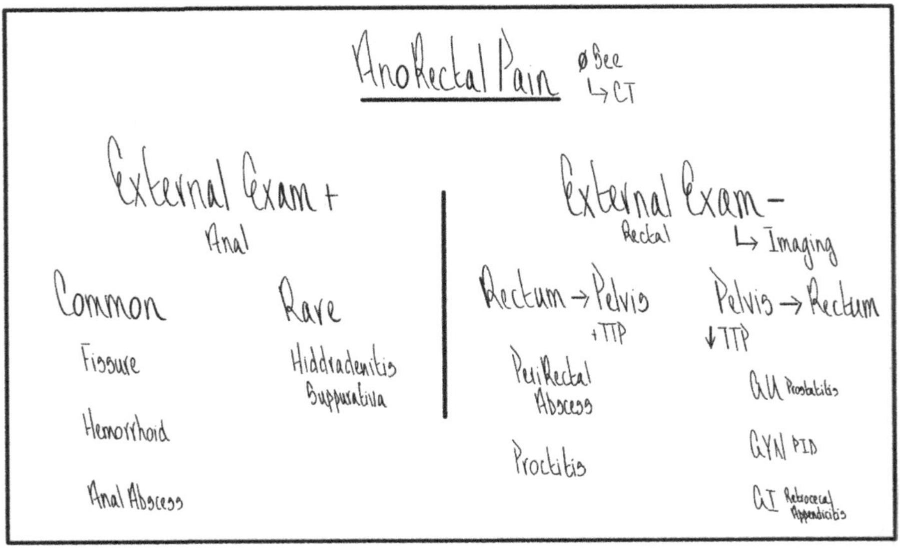

A positive external exam localizes the source; a negative exam shifts concern to deeper rectal or pelvic pathology.

Rabih adjusted the light and, just loud enough for Reza to hear, said, "Anorectal exams punish shyness."

They spread the tissue deliberately, searching folds and margins. Still nothing. With lubrication and warning, Reza attempted a digital rectal exam. The reaction was immediate. The patient recoiled, lifting off the table.

"I'm sorry. I can't." He pulled away. The pain was explosive. He reflexively expelled Reza's finger.

Pause and Reflect

What problem are you solving?

Rabih kept his voice low. "If we can't see it, it's probably inside."

The picture sharpened. This was not external pathology. This was mucosal inflammation. Pain worsening during bowel movements meant stool was aggravating inflamed rectal tissue.

Proctitis.

In a young patient without chronic gastrointestinal symptoms, infection rose quickly to the top of the list. Context mattered now. They took a sexual history carefully, not as a checkbox, but because exposure determined probability. He was sexually active with men and took HIV pre-exposure prophylaxis. His most recent HIV test one month earlier was negative. No prior known sexually transmitted infections. None of this ruled infection out, but it refined the probability.

They swabbed intentionally for rectal gonorrhea and chlamydia, syphilis, and HIV. They treated empirically with ceftriaxone and doxycycline.

"You don't wait for certainty here," Rabih said as they finalized orders.

Two days later, the patient returned.

They were again in their same seats when the triage note updated. The same chairs, the same monitors, the same hum of the department around them.

The patient was standing when they entered the exam room, bracing his hands on the edge of the bed as if sitting were no longer an option.

"My pain didn't get better." Then he hesitated, pulling up his sleeve. "And now I have this rash."

He turned slowly. Vesicles were scattered across his buttock. When he removed his shirt, papules appeared across his chest. A few lesions on his elbow and forearm looked pustular and newly evolved.

Reza exchanged a glance with Rabih.

Vesicles changed the frame, instantly widening the case. This was no longer single-organ reasoning. Distribution, timing, and epidemiology mattered.

Rash changes the diagnostic architecture.

Figure 4.2

Rash + Proctitis: Infectious vs Autoimmune

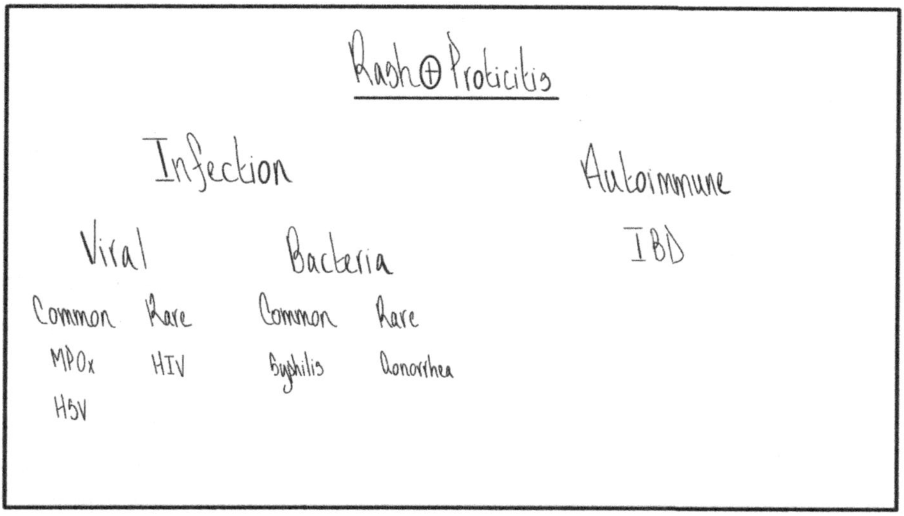

Sexually transmitted infections are the predominant cause of rash and proctitis.

Pause and Reflect

With rectal pain and a multifocal vesicular rash, what is your immediate next move?

The immediate priority was not naming the pathogen but controlling exposure. They isolated the patient, not because they were certain, but because they were not. It was done quietly, without drama, preserving dignity while protecting staff and other patients.

Back in the workroom, Reza paused, tracing the thought as it formed. "Vesicles push viral."

Rabih folded his arms loosely. “Varicella. HSV. Syphilis still fits. Autoimmune stays in the background, but infection leads.”

Results returned the next day.

Syphilis serology positive. RPR 1:64.

Rabih watched the result appear on the screen. “That fits,” he said, more to himself than anyone else.

Secondary syphilis could explain the rash and the proctitis. Syphilis, the great imitator, could move quietly as spirochetes spread from a usually painless chancre to a disseminated illness involving the skin, nervous system, gastrointestinal tract, and other organs.

What had felt diffuse and uncertain now unfurled into something actionable. They treated with intramuscular penicillin and counseled the patient about the Jarisch–Herxheimer reaction. The syndrome felt plausibly closed.

But sexually transmitted infections often traveled together. Could another diagnosis be wearing a syphilitic coat?

Then additional testing returned: *PCR for mpox, positive.*

What had seemed like a single-pathogen story now split into two. The case finally cohered, not in simplicity, but in layers.

Public health became involved. One month later, he was well.

Recap

- Pain worsened by bowel movements localizes disease to the rectal mucosa. Tenesmus is a diagnostic signal.
- Some diseases travel in clusters. Sexually transmitted infections frequently coexist, and one positive result should never end the evaluation. Rather, it reinforces the need for comprehensive testing.
- When a patient returns with new findings, it is not a failure of reasoning. Sometimes a diagnosis needs time to declare itself.

5

Rabih adjusted the pin on the chest press machine and sat down, gripping the handles with intent.

"Twenty minutes," he said. "I set a timer. Full body. That's all I've got."

This year he was building strength. Not endless cardio. Compound movements, no wasted effort.

The gym was quiet at this hour. A few treadmills were running nearby, the noise a steady whir. Somewhere in the back, a dumbbell hit rubber flooring. Rabih pressed the handles forward, controlled and deliberate.

"While I do this," the machine glided back toward his chest, "let me tell you about a thumb."

"Cold. Dark. Couldn't move it. The kind of stillness you don't get in living tissue."

He locked out the rep and exhaled.

"Gangrenous."

The patient had presented with a thumb that was black, exquisitely painful, cold, and immobile. Before debating mechanisms or naming syndromes, the first question was simple. Was it being perfused?

Doppler signals. Sensation. Motor function.

The diagnosis could wait. Tissue could not.

Rabih wiped his hands and moved to pull-ups.

"He couldn't move it. And it wasn't new. Weeks."

Weeks mattered. It felt less acute now and more like circulation fading over time.

Pause and Reflect

If you already know the diagnosis, ask us for a refund. If not, let's reflect. What is the true problem in front of us, and how do we localize it?

When a digit went cold, ischemia was the cause. But what caused ischemia?

Pump. Pipes. Plasma.

Start here.

Figure 5.1

Thrombosis Overview: Pump, Pipes, and Plasma

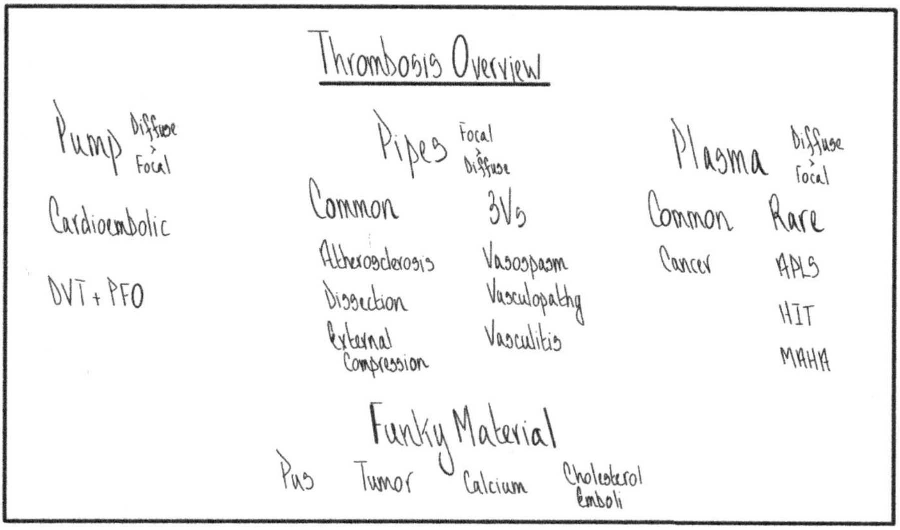

The causes of thrombosis can be categorized based on the anatomic location within the cardiovascular system.

1. *The pump.* The heart. Was it sending something forward that should not be there?

2. *The pipes.* The arteries and branches. Were they narrowed, dissected, progressively closing?

3. *The plasma.* Was the blood itself primed to clot?

But before all of that, the phenomenon must be confirmed. Was this truly ischemia?

Pause and Reflect

What are the mimics of gangrene?

Hematoma. Infection. Achenbach syndrome (whoops, we just lost you to Google, didn't we). A finger could look frightening without being threatened.

But this thumb was cold, immobile, and severely painful. This was ischemia.

Rabih dropped from the pull-up bar and rested his forearms on his thighs, breathing heavier than he wanted to admit.

"So, I asked myself, acute or chronic?"

Acute pushed toward embolism, vasospasm, and dissection. Chronic suggested progressive occlusion such as atherosclerosis, vessel-to-vessel thrombosis, or inflammatory vasculopathy.

The clinical presentation had been evolving for weeks. Weeks made an embolus unlikely, made vasospasm less convincing, and suggested a slow loss of blood flow.

Rabih moved to dumbbell presses. One set, controlled, unhurried. Reza watched him, his mouth itching to say: *that's not enough volume.* Because hypertrophy needed time under tension. It needed repetition. But that wasn't the goal, was it? The goal was the case. The goal was always the next case.

"Chronic," Rabih said between reps, pulling Reza from his reverie. "So now what?"

"Any other digits involved?"

Rabih shook his head. "Just the thumb."

Just the thumb. Single digit, small-vessel territory. That narrowed the frame dramatically, drawing a tighter circle around the many possible conclusions. Peripheral arterial disease. Diabetes. Progressive distal compromise.

Rabih paused mid-set, like he was deciding whether to say the next part or let Reza get there himself.

"There's one more detail."

He racked the weights.

"Fistula."

Whenever there was ischemia, the question became simple: was there trauma? Not just dog bites or crush injuries. Procedural trauma. *Had we done something?*

The patient had an arteriovenous fistula for dialysis.

Rabih moved to Romanian deadlifts, the bar close to his thighs, hinging slowly at the hips before standing tall again.

"Blood has choices," he told Reza. "If resistance is high in one direction, it flows elsewhere."

Pause and Reflect

At the bedside, how would you determine whether an AV fistula is stealing blood from the hand?

Blood leaving the heart traveled down the brachial artery toward the hand. At the fistula, it faced two exits. One path continued distally toward the digits. The other diverted into the vein through the fistula, an intentionally low-resistance circuit. If the distal arteries narrowed, the path to the hand carried higher resistance. The fistula's venous outflow did not carry that same resistance. Blood now had more reason to follow the easier route.

"I tested it," Rabih said, unable to hide the satisfaction in his voice.

He stopped mid-set, reached into his pocket, and pulled out his phone. "I recorded this with Mike."

On the screen, Mike, their colleague, placed his fingers over the venous limb of the fistula, gently increasing resistance. Another hand held the Doppler over the distal artery, listening.

At first there was nothing. Silence.

Then, as the compression increased, a faint sound appeared.

Thub.

Thub thub.

The signal strengthened. Distal flow returned.

Reza stared at the screen, eyebrows lifting. "Wait, that's real?"

Rabih smiled, tapping his phone to restart the video.

Reza felt that familiar jolt, the quiet awe that came when physiology stopped being theoretical and revealed itself at the bedside.

Dialysis access steal syndrome.

It occurred in roughly three percent of patients with AV fistulas. Blood flowed from the subclavian to the axillary to the brachial artery. At the fistula, it faced a fork: continue distally into the hand or divert into the low-resistance venous circuit.

In patients with diabetes and renal failure, distal arterial resistance was often high. Blood followed the path of least resistance. The hand became ischemic. Over time, tissue died. Gangrene.

Rabih completed his final repetition and rested against the rack.

"The diagnosis wasn't magic," he said.

A week earlier, he had built a schema for AV fistula complications. Steal syndrome was on that schema, though it was not the cause in his prior patient. When the thumb appeared, the path was already mapped.

The framework he had drawn the week before looked something like this.

Figure 5.2

Dialysis Access Complications: A Mechanistic Overview

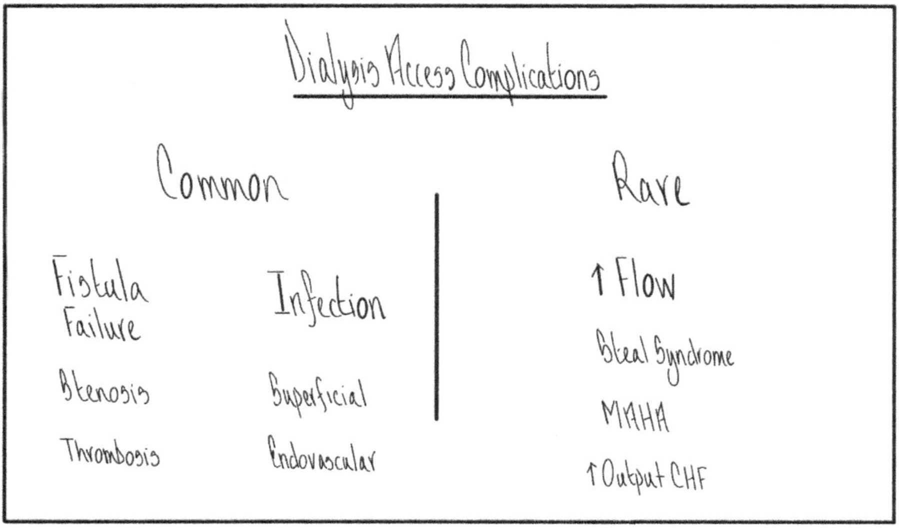

Dialysis access complications fall into predictable domains.

Tempo. Vessel size. Procedural history. Inflammation. Four structural questions that did most of the work, narrowing the frame before any imaging was ordered. A CTA was obtained to rule out large-vessel disease, but the bedside maneuver had already told the story. Vascular surgery intervened.

Rabih checked the timer. It had been nineteen minutes and thirty seconds. Full body, no wasted motion.

Strength training and diagnostic reasoning shared a rule: results followed resistance. Without deliberate schemas, cognitive energy drifted toward the easiest explanation.

The power here was not in the questions themselves but in the structure built beforehand. Once the case arrived, thinking simply mapped onto it, guiding attention to tempo, vessel size, trauma, and inflammation and forcing reasoning down more productive paths.

Rabih didn't know the diagnosis due to recall. He knew it because he had reflected the week prior, building a framework before he needed it. That was the real strength of the approach. And that preparation saved a thumb.

Recap

- Frame ischemia using a structural lens—pump, pipes, and plasma—to localize the mechanism before chasing specific diagnoses.

- Use tempo, vessel size, procedural history, and inflammatory clues as early branch points to narrow the differential before ordering tests.

6

The fluorescent lights in triage washed the room into a flat, unrelenting glow. The air carried the faint smell of worn scrubs. Nothing felt urgent enough to move quickly, and nothing felt settled enough to ignore.

"You're keeping the beard?" Rabih asked, breaking the stillness.

Reza adjusted the collar of his jacket. "You remember Arnar? Our ice cave guide in Iceland. The one who looked like he belonged in a saga."

Rabih smirked. "The Viking with the glacier beard."

"Exactly," Reza replied. "He made it look noble."

Rabih took a long look at him. "It looks anything but noble on you, my bald, beautiful man."

The jokes lingered for a beat, a fragile rhythm before the real work began. Then a new name appeared on the board. A seventy-nine-year-old man with confusion for five hours. They stood at the same time, leaving the humor behind in their chairs.

The room was dim, the blinds half drawn against the afternoon light. The patient sat upright in bed, hands resting on his thighs, as if trying to hold himself steady. His daughter hovered close, arms folded tightly across her chest, eyes moving between him and the doorway.

Reza stepped forward first. The chart stayed closed for now.

"Sir, what brings you in?"

"I feel terrible," he said.

He did not elaborate.

His daughter cut in, filling the silence. "He was normal five hours ago. But then I asked what he wanted for breakfast, and he just stared at me. Like he didn't understand the question."

His vitals were normal. A Foley catheter was in place. Blood was drawn and sent to the laboratory.

The labs returned in a few hours, one by one. White count 30,000. Neutrophils 28,000. Creatinine 2.4, up from a baseline of 0.8 just two weeks earlier. Sodium 131. Bicarbonate 18. Anion gap 21.

Then the urinalysis populated with more than one hundred white blood cells, bacteria, and cloudy urine.

Confusion plus leukocytosis plus acute kidney injury. Presumed sepsis until proven otherwise.

A bladder scan revealed six hundred milliliters of urine. The obstructed catheter was replaced, and urine poured out immediately, the tubing filling faster than expected. That kind of observation raised concern. An indwelling Foley that stopped draining could indicate an ascending infection causing obstruction, as infections could form biofilm and debris that blocked drainage.

Concern for infection prompted swift intervention. Cultures were sent. Antibiotics were started. Fluids began.

The patient had experienced this before. Two weeks earlier, he had been admitted for urinary retention and confusion. A catheter was placed. His mentation improved.

Given that history, catheter-associated urinary tract infection in the setting of obstruction became the cautious leading diagnosis. Within days, cultures grew *Klebsiella pneumoniae* in both his blood and urine. Antibiotics were narrowed. The white count fell, and the creatinine improved. His mental status cleared.

The story felt complete. Until the numbers changed.

Day one after relieving the obstruction: *6.8 liters of urine.* It did not trickle. It surged. The clear tubing filled in waves. The collection bag swelled, heavy and tense, needing to be emptied again and again.

A normal adult made one to two liters per day. Three liters defined polyuria. The patient made nearly seven.

Day two: *8.7 liters.*

Day three: *11 liters.*

Rabih stared at the output totals, the screen reflecting faintly in his glasses. "This is too much," he said, worry creeping into his voice.

Reza agreed. Some post-obstructive diuresis was expected, but this was something else entirely.

Pause and Reflect

What is the single most important test you can do on this urine, and what is the quickest way to do it?

That test was the urine osmolality, because it answered a critical question: was the kidney concentrating?

The formal measurement took time, but there was a shortcut that would give an estimate without delay. If the patient wasn't severely hyperglycemic and hadn't recently received contrast, the last two digits of the specific gravity on a simple urinalysis could be taken and multiplied by thirty. This approximated the urine osmolality.

The specific gravity was 1.001, which made the urine osmolality about 30.

Reza said their resulting thought aloud. "That's basically water."

The formal urine osmolality returned later, profoundly low, confirming what they already knew. The kidney was not retaining water.

When urine is this dilute, the diagnosis begins with classification, not labeling.

Figure 6.1

Polyuria: Solute versus Solvent Framework

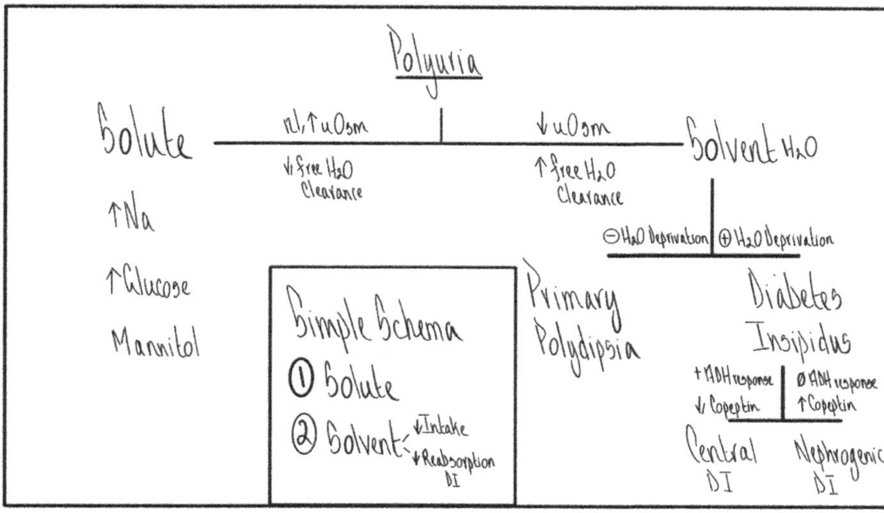

Polyuria is first classified as solute diuresis or solvent (water diuresis). The latter is then refined to determine whether a patient is drinking excessively or cannot reabsorb water in the kidney.

They moved into physiology.

Vasopressin released from the brain should signal the nephron to concentrate urine. If the urine was this dilute, either the hormone was not being released or the kidney was not responding. Diabetes insipidus entered the conversation. The frame shifted from infection to water balance.

Then a detail resurfaced.

During the patient's prior admission, an MRI had mentioned a prominent sella. Follow-up imaging had been recommended but not yet done.

As the urine output roared, the image lingered quietly in the background. Central diabetes insipidus; nephrogenic diabetes insipidus. Both remained possible.

Once diabetes insipidus enters the frame, the next move is to determine whether the problem lies in hormone production or renal response.

Figure 6.2

Central and Nephrogenic Diabetes Insipidus

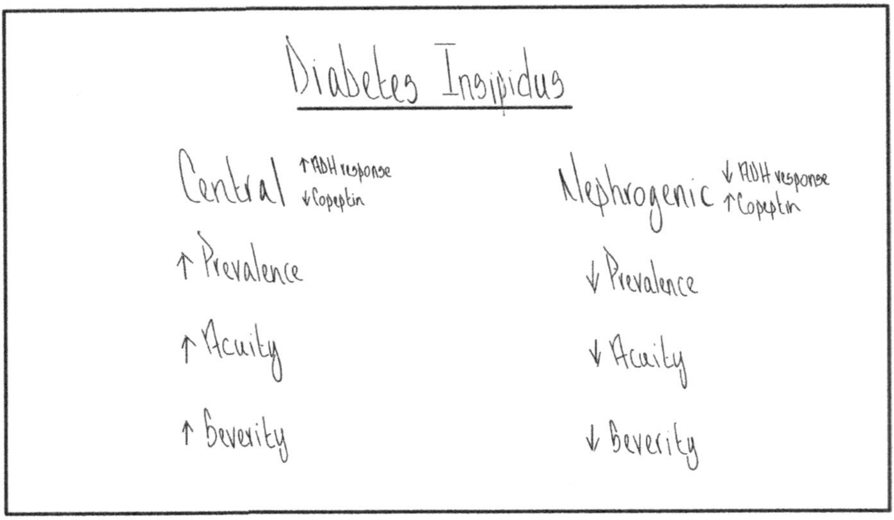

Central diabetes insipidus reflects inadequate vasopressin release; nephrogenic diabetes insipidus reflects renal resistance to vasopressin.

Reza felt the pull toward the MRI. "What if this was central all along?"

Rabih shook his head slightly. "Maybe. But look at the sequence."

The diuresis had begun *after* relieving the obstruction.

Post-obstructive states could temporarily impair the kidney's ability to respond to vasopressin. The collecting duct forgot how to listen. It mimicked diabetes insipidus even when ADH was present.

The timeline favored the kidney. Still, the MRI sat there, tempting.

Pause and Reflect

With a pituitary abnormality in the background and profound polyuria in the foreground, what would you do next?

The next step was to return to the bedside to perform examinations and to order select labs. The visual fields were intact, with no bitemporal loss. Anterior pituitary hormones were normal; cortisol and thyroid function were appropriate. The posterior pituitary could still be involved, but the probability diminished.

Meanwhile, the patient's urine continued to pour out. The steady drainage became a background noise in his room.

Rabih suggested matching every liter with IV fluid.

Reza hesitated. "If we keep replacing it aggressively, we might perpetuate this."

They monitored the sodium closely and watched the trajectory of urine output. Over the next forty-eight hours, the numbers shifted: eleven liters became four, then three, then two.

Specific gravity rose. The kidney remembered how to concentrate. The storm passed without desmopressin.

The MRI abnormality was visible, tangible, satisfying. It offered a clean explanation. But coherence, however compelling, was not synonymous with truth.

The patient completed treatment for *Klebsiella* bacteremia and urinary tract infection. Creatinine returned to baseline, sodium remained stable, and the urine output normalized. The outpatient pituitary protocol MRI eventually revealed a 1.7-centimeter macroadenoma—a finding that rarely caused diabetes insipidus.

Two truths could coexist. An image could be important and irrelevant at the same time.

Recap

- Polyuria begins with specific gravity. In someone who is not having primary polydipsia, when the urine is profoundly dilute, the frame becomes central versus nephrogenic diabetes insipidus.

- Understanding the sequence of events is a powerful diagnostic tool: what happened first and what followed?

- Radiographic findings can be real yet incidental. That is why radiology reports say, "correlate clinically," and a safeguard is to call a finding radiographic until it clearly maps onto a clinical syndrome or is confirmed by pathology.

7

Rabih, you are not going to believe this diagnosis.

Reza told Rabih that on the second tee box.

Rabih had shown up that morning shaking his head. "It's my day off. I don't even play golf." And after a beat: "You owe me for this."

Reza promised him it would be fun. He didn't tell him that a case would follow them onto the course.

They were paired with two retirees who played slowly, spoke rarely, and hit every fairway. Fog lifted in thin sheets off the grass. Reza's phone rested in the cupholder of the pushcart, face down, and he kept glancing at it.

"You think you've got liver tests all figured out," Reza said as he lined up his shot, "then a case shakes things up. This one basically debunked something we learned back in med school."

Rabih squinted at him. "Bit dramatic."

"You know how we're taught the liver is hard to infarct because of its dual blood supply?"

"That's the teaching."

Reza swung the driver. It leaked right. Not disastrous, not good.

"Sixty-two-year-old man," he continued as they started walking. "Five days of waxing and waning right upper quadrant pain. Febrile to 102°F. AST 92. ALT 61. Total bilirubin 3.2. Alk phos 286."

Rabih nodded. "Fever plus cholestasis is cholangitis until proven otherwise."

"Exactly. So we treated it like cholangitis. Blood cultures. Fluids. Broad gram-negative and anaerobic coverage. GI consult. MRCP ordered."

Reza found his ball in the rough.

"An ultrasound showed stones but no biliary dilatation. CT showed no dilated ducts. No dramatic hepatic abnormality. Possible early diverticulitis in the left lower quadrant."

"He had left lower quadrant pain?"

"None."

Rabih took his swing. It was the dreaded slice of a beginner: a sharp, violent arc to the right. The sight brought an unkind sense of satisfaction to Reza: Rabih was finally failing at something in front of him.

Rabih shrugged, already walking, already back in the case.

"Five days matters," he shared as they pushed the cart up the fairway. "Cholangitis usually declares itself faster. That tempo lowers confidence but doesn't erase the diagnosis."

"That's what unsettled me."

By the time they reached the green, Reza had told him what changed the case last week.

"The MRCP came back without biliary dilatation," he explained. "Instead, it showed a wedge-shaped lesion in the right hepatic lobe, suspicious for infarct."

The LDH was 450.

Rabih studied Reza's face, his expression inscrutable. "What?"

"Hepatic infarct," he said.

Rabih exhaled through his nose. "I've never seen one."

"Me neither."

The retirees putted in silence. The wind held steady.

"The liver has dual blood supply," Rabih stated. "Hepatic artery. Portal vein. It's hard to infarct."

"That's the teaching," Reza replied, echoing Rabih's earlier words.

Rabih started solving. "Treat it like a stroke in an organ. Two questions. Where did the occlusion occur, and what's the material? We default to a bland clot. But fever forces us to consider an infected clot. Pus can occlude just as effectively as fibrin."

They walked to the next tee.

"A Doppler ultrasound came next," Reza said. "Portal vein thrombosis involving the right portal venous system. Triple-phase CT confirmed complete occlusion of the right portal vein, including anterior and posterior branches, tracking to the wedge-shaped lesion."

Rabih shook his head. "Now the fork. Bland or infected?"

Reza smiled. That was why he brought Rabih golfing.

Because he always saw the fork.

Pause and Reflect

What is the most common cause of portal vein thrombosis, and what other etiologies should you consider?

Once thrombosis is identified, the task becomes etiologic sorting.

Figure 7.1

Portal Vein Thrombosis: Etiologic Categories

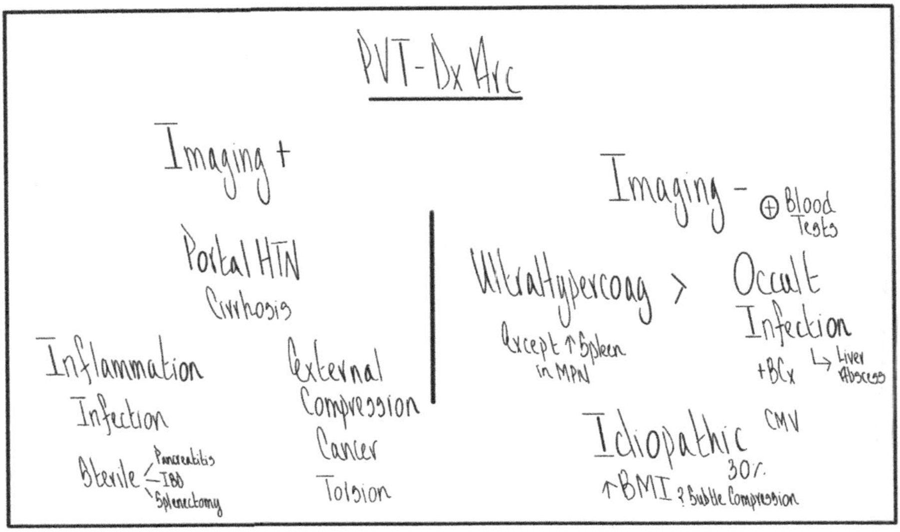

Imaging is a key tool to study the causes of portal vein thrombosis. The most common cause is cirrhosis.

Rabih didn't hesitate.

"Most portal vein thromboses are bland clots. And most of those are from cirrhosis."

"He doesn't have cirrhosis."

"Then we're in the non-cirrhotic bucket."

He teed up his ball.

"Next comes abdominal malignancy and inflammation. Hepatocellular carcinoma. Pancreatic cancer. IBD. Pancreatitis. Anything local that can irritate the portal system."

"And if there's no obvious inflammation?" Reza asked.

Rabih looked up. "Systemic hypercoagulability. Myeloproliferative neoplasms. JAK2 mutations. They favor the splanchnic veins."

"But here's the tension. He's febrile beyond what mild abdominal inflammation should cause."

Rabih made another terrible swing, barely making contact with the ball, and glanced at Reza without an ounce of shame.

"Fever changes the clot," he said. "Now we have to consider that it's not bland at all. It could be infected."

The fog had burned off by then, leaving the course quiet and bright.

On the seventh hole, Reza's phone buzzed. He grabbed it from the pushcart, unlocking it hastily.

It was the patient's primary care physician.

The message read: *One of four blood culture bottles is growing Fusobacterium.*

Reza stopped walking.

Rabih took a few steps before he noticed. He turned. "What?"

"*Fusobacterium.*"

Pause and Reflect

What is the final diagnosis? After diagnosing it, what investigation is essential?

Rabih smiled slowly.

"Bacteremia plus thrombosis isn't noise."

Before naming a diagnosis, we localize infection within the liver itself, parenchyma, or plumbing.

Figure 7.2

Hepatic Infection: Localizing Parenchyma Versus Plumbing

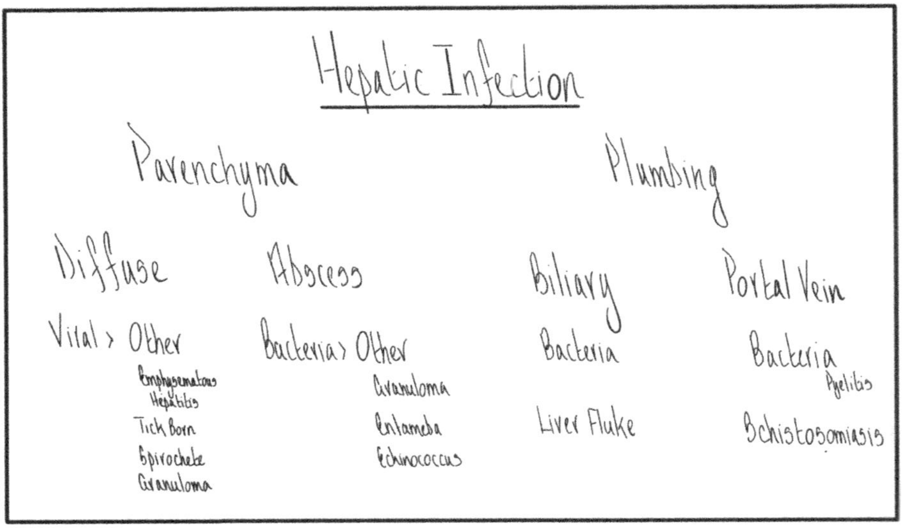

Liver infection may involve the parenchyma (diffuse hepatitis or focal abscess) or the biliary and portal venous systems.

"Pylephlebitis," Reza said. "Infected portal vein thrombosis. An abdominal variant of Lemierre syndrome."

They stood in the fairway, neither of them caring about the score.

"I almost stopped when he improved," Reza admitted, voice quiet. "By day three he was afebrile and comfortable. Cultures were negative then. We stopped antibiotics and discharged him on apixaban."

Rabih let out a slow breath. "Getting better can trick you."

Infectious disease later recommended a month of amoxicillin-clavulanate, and anticoagulation was continued. Because *Fusobacterium* bacteremia raised concern for a mucosal breach in the colon, including occult malignancy, a colonoscopy was required to evaluate for an anatomic source. It showed diverticular disease but no malignancy.

The patient completed therapy. Liver tests normalized, and portal flow improved. He felt well.

On the eighteenth green, Rabih asked, "So what did it debunk?"

"That the liver can't infarct unless both blood supplies fail."

He shook his head. "Dual supply lowers risk. It doesn't eliminate it."

Reza tapped in for par.

What stayed with him wasn't that he named pylephlebitis immediately. He hadn't. They empirically treated cholangitis because missing it would have been catastrophic. They escalated imaging, questioned the clot, and followed the data, even after discharge. The diagnosis came because they hadn't stopped asking.

He wasn't ashamed of that. Medicine wasn't about hitting it pure on the first swing. It was about how you recovered from the shot that went astray.

Recap

- When a potentially life-threatening diagnosis such as cholangitis is plausible, lower your threshold to treat early because the cost of delay might be the difference between life and death.
- When you identify an infarct, ask where the occlusion occurred and what the occluding material is, because that distinction directs the diagnostic and therapeutic strategy.
- Fever in the setting of thrombosis should prompt consideration of an infected clot and a deliberate search for an anatomic source of bacteremia.

8

Rabih and Reza stood outside the patient's room, the electronic chart already open between them.

Reza shifted his coffee to the other hand, steam curling off the top. "Still making your own açaí?"

"If I don't make it, I don't eat it," Rabih said, a touch defensive.

The screen pulled them back.

CT images glowed against the dim workstation light: *left lower lobe consolidation, a small effusion, pleural thickening.* Rabih scrolled through the prior scans. Same location, same density. Six weeks earlier.

Reza leaned in, tracing the timeline. "Two courses of antibiotics…"

"And it's still there," Rabih said, tapping the screen.

Reza took a slow sip of coffee, eyes still fixed on the image. "Six weeks is long, right?"

"No question. So what are we calling this?"

"Doesn't feel like simple pneumonia."

"No," Rabih exhaled through his nose. "If it were, it should've cleared by now."

"Or at least improved," Reza added.

They let the image sit there for a moment longer. Persistence was no longer treatment failure. It was diagnostic signal.

That thought stayed with them as they entered the room. The patient was sitting upright when they walked in, back straight, shoulders held as if he refused to sink into the stiff hospital bed. He looked up when they introduced themselves and offered a small acknowledgement in return.

"I'm just tired," he said once the pleasantries were over. The exhaustion in his voice preceded his words. "These fevers never stop."

"How high do they get?" Reza asked, stepping nearer to the bedside.

The patient seemed to search for the answer through his fog of fatigue. "One-oh-two. Sometimes higher. I wake up drenched."

His wife sat quietly in the corner, looking anxious as she watched him endure another bout of fever.

"He changes his shirt twice a night," she told them. "He's never been like this."

They pulled up chairs.

"When did you last feel normal?" Rabih prompted.

The patient let out a long, slow exhale. "Before all this. Before they said pneumonia. But I took the antibiotics. I did everything."

Six weeks of recurrent fevers, night sweats, and twenty pounds lost. Two antibiotic courses. A left lower lobe opacity that never fully cleared. The fevers had subsided, then returned.

"Shortness of breath?"

"No."

"Cough?"

"Not really. A little in the mornings maybe."

His vitals revealed a temperature of 101.5°F, a heart rate of 110, and stable blood pressure and oxygenation. No respiratory distress. No shock. No hypoxemia. No airway compromise. That bought time to think.

When a consolidation refuses to clear, the question shifts from treatment to mechanism.

Figure 8.1

Persistent Pulmonary Opacity: Pneumonia Mimics

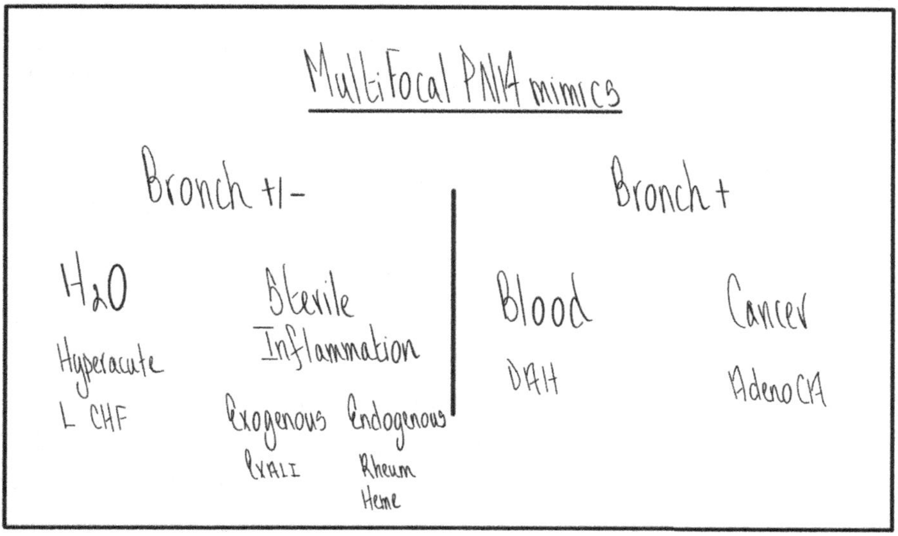

Infectious, malignant, inflammatory, vascular, and hemorrhagic processes can all mimic pneumonia radiographically. A bronchoscopy is a valuable tool to sift through this differential diagnosis.

Pause and Reflect

How are you framing this patient?

Tempo mattered. This was not acute or chronic over years. It was subacute. Six weeks of inflammatory weight loss, fevers, and persistent consolidation. ESR and CRP elevated. Ferritin 1200.

Rabih named the frame aloud. "Subacute inflammatory thoracic syndrome with pleuroparenchymal involvement."

Naming the problem narrowed the path. Inflammatory weight loss created three broad buckets: infection, malignancy, and autoimmune disease. Autoimmune disease drifted lower on the differential. No rash, no arthritis, no renal involvement. That left infection and malignancy. Chronic unilateral consolidation with pleural thickening narrowed it further. Adenocarcinoma. Lymphoma. Granulomatous infection.

The patient worked in construction on the East Coast. Construction exposed workers to soil and dust where fungal spores lived, organisms that could cause subacute pneumonia after inhalation.

The infectious workup returned negative. Blood cultures, fungal studies, rickettsial serologies. Nothing.

Next, a PET-CT was obtained, revealing more of the story. Hypermetabolic mediastinal and hilar nodes, upper abdominal lymphadenopathy, left adrenal uptake, and a lytic iliac lesion. This was no longer a pneumonia that refused to resolve.

The findings leaned toward malignancy. The adrenal uptake whispered cancer. The IgG lambda nudged toward hematologic disease.

But paraproteins were suggestive, not declarative. MGUS could coexist by chance. Lymphoma could mimic almost anything.

The iliac bone lesion was biopsied. Benign chondromyxoid fibroma. Bone marrow normal. For a moment, it became clear how close they had come to forcing a single narrative. They had incorrectly assumed that everything belonged to one disease. It didn't. Not every abnormality deserved membership in the same explanation.

They returned to the bedside before planning another procedure.

"We still don't have an answer," Reza began, his tone apologetic.

The patient gave a faint acknowledgment. His wife leaned forward, frowning. "Another procedure?"

"The lung is one option," Rabih replied. "But the lymph nodes are safer. If this is systemic, they may tell us more."

The patient looked between them—the doctors and his wife. "Do what you need to do."

A lymph node was biopsied.

Non-caseating granulomas.

Pause and Reflect

What is your differential diagnosis?

A granuloma is not a diagnosis. It is an immune pattern.

Figure 8.2

Granuloma: Mechanistic Differential

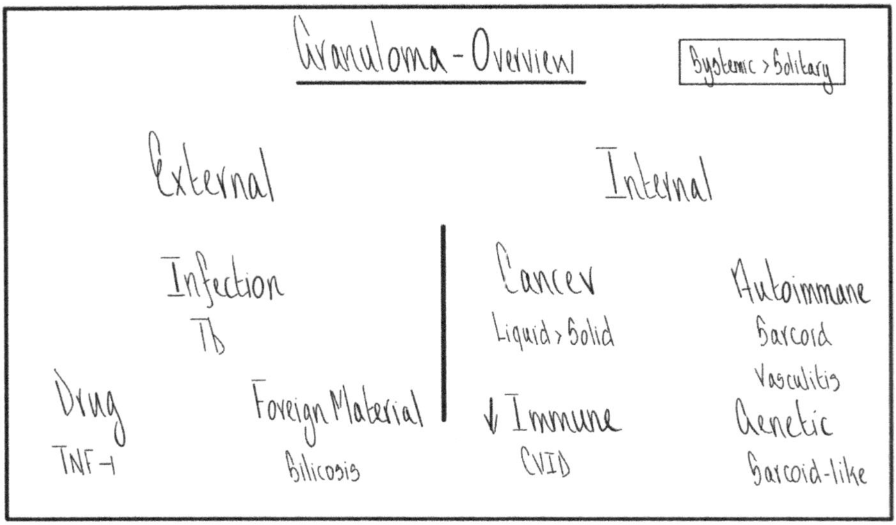

Granulomas represent organized immune responses to persistent antigenic stimulation, which is usually external but may also come from inside the body.

Granulomas shortened the list. Infection. Sarcoidosis. Lymphoma masquerading.

Infection had been aggressively pursued and remained unrevealing. Malignancy showed no evidence on biopsy. Sarcoidosis began to rise. But sarcoidosis with unilateral consolidation and pleural effusion was uncommon.

Rabih leaned back in their shared workroom. “Illness scripts are guides. Not rules.”

Reza added, “Diseases aren’t obligated to follow their chapter in a textbook.”

Pause and Reflect

When a biopsy shows non-caseating granulomas, do you accept sarcoidosis or continue searching for cancer?

They did both, but sarcoidosis carried the strongest explanatory power. Vigilance remained, however. Fifteen percent of patients initially labeled with sarcoid later proved to have lymphoma.

The patient improved over the next few days. His fevers subsided.

They favored sarcoidosis. The granulomas and systemic pattern fit. But the picture was suggestive, not sealed. So they did not begin immunosuppression. Infection had been pursued, malignancy sampled, but certainty in medicine was rarely declared in a single stroke.

So, they watched.

A week later, the board lit up with the patient's name once more. Eye pain and blurry vision.

Rabih and Reza saw him in the emergency department. His left eye was red and photophobic. The slit lamp exam confirmed anterior uveitis. They looked at each other before either of them spoke. The final piece slid into place.

Sarcoidosis.

"So, that's what it is," the patient said calmly, as if something had finally settled.

"Yes," Rabih answered. "It explains the lungs, the nodes, the eyes."

His wife, hovering nearby, asked, "It's not cancer?"

"No," Reza said, his tone certain.

The patient was started on methotrexate for symptomatic sarcoidosis and improved shortly after. His chest imaging cleared.

Oftentimes, in medicine, there was discipline in saying, “We don’t know yet,” and waiting long enough for the body to finish the sentence.

Recap

- The most important step in diagnosis is framing the problem correctly, and challenging cases often require reframing as new data emerges.
- Diseases frequently deviate from textbook presentations, so illness scripts must remain flexible when patterns stretch.
- Protect trust by openly communicating uncertainty.

9

A monitor chirped nearby, and a stretcher rattled past. Rabih turned his phone toward Reza, a grin already tugging at his lips.

"Naar learned a new trick," he said.

On the screen, his dog appeared frozen midair, all four paws off the ground, ears flopping like tiny wings—pure joy captured in a single frame. Rabih looked delighted, nudging the phone closer to Reza as if to say, *see? Impossible not to love this.*

Reza shook his head, smiling.

They were finishing a note, still half laughing at the photo, when a nurse walked by.

"Room 7 is here with hiccups," he mentioned in passing.

They looked up.

"Hiccups?"

A glance passed between them. A small smile. A tiny wrinkle of confusion. Hiccups plagued everyone—the universal annoyance, the body's little glitch. But neither of them had cared for a patient who came to the emergency department because they could not stop. It felt almost trivial. And yet, the nurse's tone suggested otherwise.

They stood and started toward the room.

"Do you actually have an approach to hiccups?" Rabih asked, tipping his head the way Naar sometimes did.

Reza thought for a moment.

"Honestly? No. Hold your breath. Drink water. Get startled." A beat, then, "That's the full extent of my medical training, courtesy of my mom."

Rabih laughed. "Same."

Then they stepped inside.

The patient sat upright in the bed, her husband close beside her. Sixty-nine years old. Kind face, calm eyes. Every few seconds, her body jerked forward, interrupting itself as if on an irrationally timed schedule. Her husband reached over and rubbed her back each time, the way you did when there was nothing else to do.

"I'm Dr. Rabih, and this is Dr. Reza," Rabih said, with the easy manner he'd walked in wearing. "We usually go by our first names. Our last names have been creatively interpreted over the years."

A small laugh moved through the room. The air loosened.

"It just won't stop," the husband said, his voice pitching down to a soothing lull. "She can barely sleep."

The patient started to speak, offering a small, embarrassed smile. "I don't even—"

Hic.

She closed her eyes briefly.

"She's tried everything," her husband continued. "Holding her breath, drinking water, sugar. Nothing works."

Rabih and Reza exchanged a look: curious, uncertain, already hooked. They had entered expecting triviality. They were already revising that assessment.

Seven days, the patient told them. Day and night without relief.

Pause and Reflect

How do you approach persistent hiccups?

They did not have an approach to hiccups. So they did the sensible thing: they slowed down.

They examined her from head to toe, unhurried, looking for anything that did not fit. For a moment, they felt like interns again. That particular mix of humility and intrigue, starting from scratch because there was nowhere else to start from.

Her vitals were normal. She had walked in on her own, which reassured them. Neurologic exam nonfocal. Strength full in all four extremities, no sensory deficits. Breathing comfortably.

They moved methodically, making their way down. Then they reached the abdomen. Her left upper quadrant was tender to palpation. Not spontaneous pain, not something she'd come in complaining about. She hadn't noticed it before.

They stepped back and summarized aloud. *Persistent hiccups, seven days. Normal vitals. Nonfocal neuro exam. Left upper quadrant tenderness, exam-elicited, new.*

Labs returned a few hours later. One number immediately grabbed their attention.

White blood cell count: 15,000.

But it was the differential that mattered more. Ninety percent lymphocytes, hemoglobin normal, platelets normal. Electrolytes and renal function normal. LDH mildly elevated.

A high lymphocyte count demands structure.

Figure 9.1

Lymphocytosis: Polyclonal vs. Monoclonal

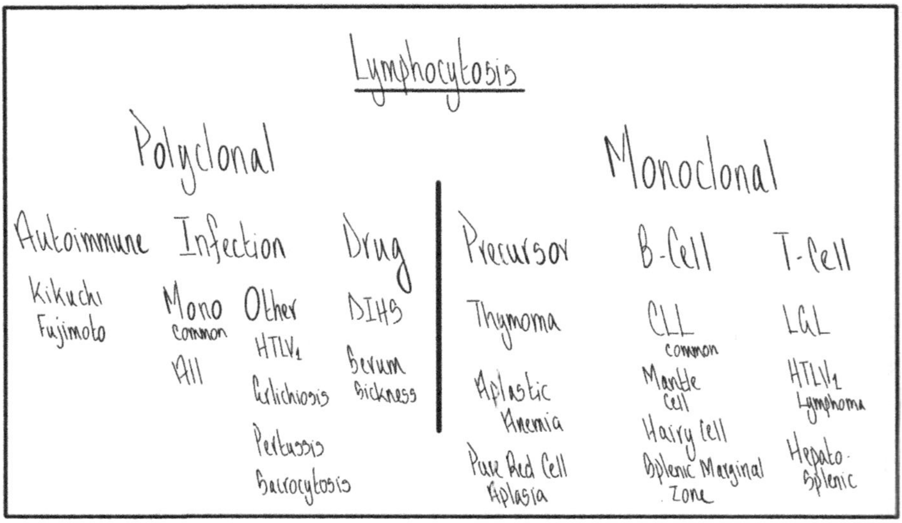

Age, tempo, associated cytopenias, lymphadenopathy, and splenomegaly help distinguish benign infection from hematologic malignancy.

Pause and Reflect

With lymphocytosis, LUQ pain, and hiccups, what are you worried about, and what focused physical examination must you perform?

They returned to the bedside with a different agenda. This wasn't about a number. It was about anatomy.

Rabih palpated the left upper quadrant slowly and deliberately. Then he moved to the cervical chains, the axillae, the inguinal regions. Small, mobile lymph nodes emerged under his fingers. Subtle, but real.

The patient felt well. No weight loss, no fevers, no night sweats. But the laboratory abnormality now had a physical counterpart.

Stepping out once more, they recognized that the situation had evolved.

Persistent hiccups. Left upper quadrant tenderness. Lymphocytosis. Diffuse small lymphadenopathy.

"This changes everything," Rabih murmured.

They started thinking in buckets: viral syndromes, medication-related causes, hematologic malignancy.

Infectious mononucleosis caused by EBV or CMV was the most common viral cause for lymphadenopathy and lymphocytosis. But she lacked symptoms such as fever, pharyngitis, or fatigue.

Drug-induced hypersensitivity syndrome was unlikely, as she was not taking any known offending medications such as allopurinol and did not have other features of the syndrome, including fever, rash, facial edema, or eosinophilia.

That left malignancy, and here, the pieces started pulling in one direction. Her age, the lymphocytosis, the nodes. Chronic lymphocytic leukemia quickly rose to the top of the differential.

They pulled prior labs. Subtle lymphocytosis had been sitting there for years, never quite enough to trigger alarm. Never enough to change the frame.

Imaging was the next step. The chest X-ray came back first: clear, unremarkable. A small exhale, then back to waiting.

They were standing at their workstation, side by side, when the CT abdomen returned. Rabih scrolled slowly, and Reza leaned in, one hand braced on the desk.

The spleen was massive. And near the dome, abutting the diaphragm, sat a wedge-shaped infarct.

They paused together, staring at the image. Now the pieces connected. The spleen had been slowly enlarging over years, outgrowing its blood supply. Until a portion infarcted. The infarct pressed against the diaphragm, and the diaphragm was made irritable.

A hiccup was simply a rapid involuntary contraction of the diaphragm. If irritation persisted, the reflex persisted. The spleen was the trigger. The hiccups were the clue. Chronic lymphocytic leukemia with massive splenomegaly and splenic infarction causing diaphragmatic irritation and persistent hiccups. In a patient who just wanted to sleep at night.

She was admitted that evening, and treatment began. The hiccups slowly faded.

A few days later, Rabih and Reza sat side by side in the Manhattan Beach Library, the Pacific stretching wide and flat beyond the windows. Rabih had a notebook open. Reza was scrolling through research articles on his laptop, occasionally turning the screen to present something particularly interesting.

Outside, the city was bright and unbothered in its usual sun-washed ease. But in here, the world narrowed to the two of them and a case that hadn't fully let go yet.

"Let's start from first principles," Reza said, eyes still on his computer. "What actually is a hiccup?"

It was a reflex arc. An afferent limb: vagus nerve, sympathetic chain, phrenic nerve. A central processor in the brainstem. Then an efferent limb. The phrenic nerve fired, the diaphragm contracted, air rushed in, and the glottis snapped shut.

Hic.

Anything that irritated any part of the arc—brainstem, neck, mediastinum, stomach, liver, spleen, diaphragm—could trigger repetitive firing. If hiccups lasted less than forty-eight hours, they were usually benign. If they persisted, the question became anatomical. What was irritating the arc?

If it is a reflex, it can be localized.

Figure 9.2

Persistent Hiccups: Localizing Along the Reflex Arc

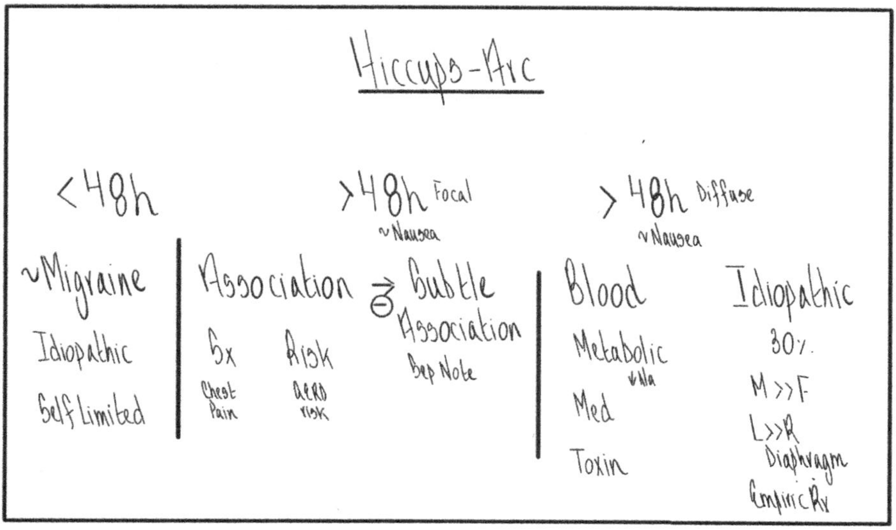

Duration helps guide evaluation: episodes under 48 hours are usually benign; persistent hiccups warrant an anatomic search along the arc. If none is found, the problem is in the blood or may never be fully understood.

They had walked into the patient's room without an approach. They walked out with something harder to name: a sharper eye, refined curiosity, and less certainty about what a complaint could or couldn't mean.

Recap

- It is okay not to have an approach at first. Be honest about what you don't know. The only real mistake is facing the same problem twice and not improving the second time.

- Use duration and the reflex arc to guide evaluation. Hiccups lasting less than forty-eight hours are usually benign; persistent hiccups should prompt an anatomic search along the reflex pathway from brainstem to diaphragm.

- Let new data reframe the problem. What began as hiccups became lymphocytosis, lymphadenopathy, splenomegaly, and ultimately chronic lymphocytic leukemia. Revisiting the exam and updating the frame changed the course of the case.

10

The emergency department was one person short. Rabih studied the board. Reza studied Rabih.

Then an ambulance pulled into the bay. A patient was wheeled in, sitting upright on the stretcher. He held two canes like briefcases, knuckles tight around the handles.

"I'm here because you people didn't give me my insulin last time," he said sharply. "And you refused my oxycodone."

EMS reported a field glucose of 512; in the ED, it was 497. Vitals were normal. He looked angry, not sick.

Rabih turned towards Reza, speaking quietly. "Easy one."

Reza paused. "That's exactly what makes it dangerous."

Pause and Reflect

What are the two hyperglycemic emergencies you need to rule out, and how do they differ?

They screened for diabetic ketoacidosis (DKA) and hyperosmolar hyperglycemic state (HHS).

Both reflected insulin deficiency, but not equally. In DKA, the absence of insulin permitted ketone production and acidosis, which often declared itself early with abdominal pain and vomiting and brought patients to care before the glucose could dramatically rise. In HHS, residual insulin suppressed ketosis but not hyperglycemia, allowing glucose to rise unchecked and osmotic diuresis to progress. This led to profound dehydration and a more insidious presentation, sometimes with altered mental status.

Severe hyperglycemia is not a number. It is a risk state with predictable patterns of injury.

Figure 10

Hyperglycemia: Organizing Acute and End-Organ Complications

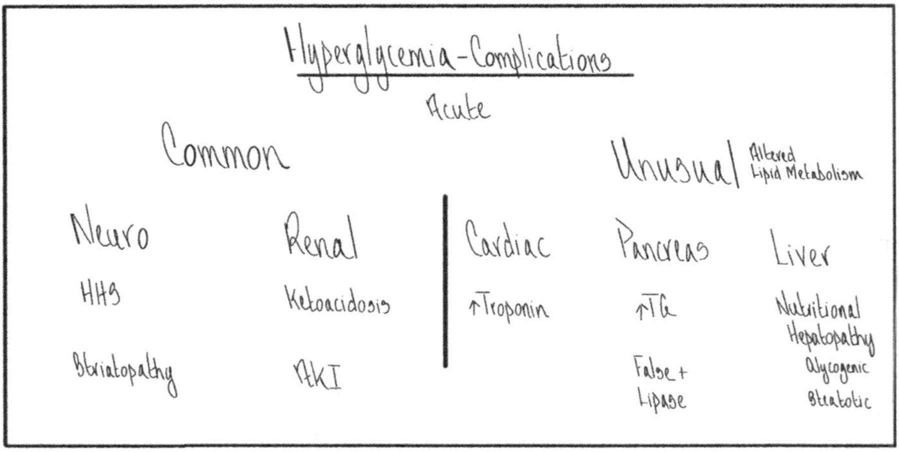

Acute hyperglycemia may present as diabetic ketoacidosis or a hyperosmolar hyperglycemic state, but sustained elevation also produces renal, neurologic, cardiac, pancreatic, and hepatic complications.

Pause and Reflect

What one question, one physical exam finding, and one lab would you obtain to ensure the patient is not in a hyperglycemic emergency?

They asked about abdominal pain, which was often the visceral hallmark of DKA. They watched the respiratory rate, looking for increased respirations. And they ordered a BMP with attention to the bicarbonate and anion gap.

Then they started fluids because most people at a glucose of 500 were dry even when they looked comfortable.

And they refused to let a refill request distract them from metabolic risk.

The patient was not tachypneic. No abdominal pain. He was oriented to person, place, and time.

"See," Rabih commented, "just hyperglycemia."

But Reza felt a small friction. It was not the patient's anger. They saw anger every shift. It was the misalignment. The intensity of his anger did not match the simplicity of his request.

Rabih opened the chart. The patient had longstanding insulin dependence with A1Cs in the double digits for years. Oxycodone for severe peripheral arterial disease, multiple revascularizations, low-dose plan. Then Rabih scrolled. Eight ED visits in the last month.

Reza exhaled, reading over Rabih's shoulder. "That's not noise."

Rabih acknowledged him. "That's signal."

They read the most recent note. *Insulin refilled. Opioids not refilled due to contract. PCP notified.* Thoughtful documentation from a colleague they both respected. Rabih clicked out of the chart without saying anything more.

They returned to the bedside soon after. The patient sat the way he'd arrived, canes balanced across his knees, jaw set.

"They gave you insulin last time."

"No," he answered, looking indignant. "They didn't."

They could have argued, defended the chart, concluded nonadherence. But they paused instead. They questioned the brain.

Reza pulled up a chair and sat down, bringing himself level with the patient. "When were you last here?"

"Recently."

"You've been here eight times this month."

He looked startled, eyebrows lifting. "Eight? No way. Maybe two or three."

Reza let the silence sit for a moment, then spoke again. His tone was soft rather than accusatory. "Who's been helping you at home?"

"My family."

Rabih stepped closer, hands loose at his sides. "What kinds of things do they help with?"

"Food. Stuff like that."

"What are their names?"

The patient stared at a point beyond them, expression darkening. "I don't want to get into that."

The answers were not evasive. They were untethered. Rabih and Reza excused themselves quietly, stepping into the corridor.

A colleague who knew nearly every regular by name was walking past with a stethoscope tucked under one arm. He slowed when he saw them.

"How's he doing?"

"Not well," Rabih responded, looking over one shoulder in the direction of the patient. "He doesn't remember things."

The colleague stopped walking. "That's new."

It landed the way simple things did when they changed the shape of something. No longer were they treating a difficult patient. Now they were treating a difficult problem.

So they reentered the room and performed the exam they almost skipped.

The patient was alert and oriented. Remote memory was intact, though recent recall proved unreliable. Bilateral end-gaze nystagmus, finger-to-nose smooth, no appendicular ataxia.

"Stand up for me," Rabih requested.

The patient planted both canes on the linoleum floor and rose. The sway came immediately, wide and truncal, and he caught himself hard on the handles.

Pause and Reflect

Localize the site of neuropathology.

"Midline," Rabih said softly. The cerebellar vermis.

They finished the exam methodically. Strength intact, lungs clear. No focal weakness. Then Reza noticed the scar across the man's abdomen.

The scar was long and well-healed, slicing from the sternum to the navel. The patient watched him look at it but said nothing.

They left the patient's room and walked through the emergency department. The air felt particularly stiff, threaded with the smell of disinfectant and synthetic, plastic tubing.

Once in their workspace, Rabih slid into a chair and clicked into the chart. The screen's glow flattened everything into clean lines and data. He scrolled further back than before, Reza hovering over his shoulder and reading aloud.

"Gastrectomy. Pancreatectomy. Duodenal GIST."

Reza stopped reading, straightening from Rabih's shoulder. The patient's diabetes was not progressive. It was surgical, a consequence of resected anatomy.

The frame reorganized. This was not hyperglycemia and frustration. This was hyperglycemia in a nutritionally vulnerable patient with subacute cognitive decline and truncal ataxia.

Pause and Reflect

What is your next diagnostic step, and what is the most likely diagnosis?

They ordered an MRI brain with and without contrast. Out loud, they said they were ruling out stroke. Privately, they knew they were mapping a syndrome, tracing something that hadn't fully clicked into place.

The scan took two hours. In the meantime, the department moved around them, creating a steady hum of bodies and sound. They saw other patients, answered other questions, and signed other orders.

They were in the workroom once more when the radiologist called.

"Symmetric signal changes," the voice rang through. "In the thalamus, hypothalamus, and mammillary bodies."

Reza looked up. Rabih looked at Reza.

"Mammillary bodies," Reza echoed quietly.

The diagnosis came into focus: thiamine deficiency causing Wernicke encephalopathy.

It wasn't the stereotypical story of alcohol use and thiamine deficiency. Instead, the case stemmed from a history of gastrectomy, a low BMI, months without supplementation, and social isolation. A slow cognitive unraveling, documented across ten visits but never synthesized.

The patient was where they'd left him when they reentered the room. He was staring in a blank sort of way at a monitor, its steady beep droning quietly in the background. He looked up when they came in.

They pulled chairs close, meeting his gaze. He still looked guarded, like the type of person that learned to be wary of the world.

They asked him about vitamins first. He hadn't taken them in months. *Couldn't keep track,* he said, then didn't elaborate.

Then they asked about his home life, more gently than they had earlier. The electricity had been shut off. There was an eviction notice. Neighbors had reported wandering in the hallways. He told them this in a flat, even tone.

They thanked him and stepped out.

In the hallway, Rabih stopped walking, leaning against a wall. "I saw him twice. Gave insulin. Sent him home."

"Me too," Reza replied.

They stood there for a moment. Eight visits. The patient had come in eight separate times, and no one had thought to check his cognitive function.

They solved the problem in front of them instead of defining the one that mattered. Insulin and oxycodone became anchors. Once anchored, everything else blurred.

The system could produce an MRI in two hours. But it struggled to recognize a trajectory across eight encounters.

Rabih pushed himself off the wall. They had already lost enough time. IV thiamine was started. Five hundred milligrams, no more delay. In this syndrome, time was neurons.

The patient was admitted. He received nutrition, social work, medication reconciliation, and primary care reengagement. A second chance at continuity.

Later, again in the hallway, Rabih stopped Reza with a hand on his forearm.

"How do we get better at defining the problem sooner?"

Reza didn't answer right away. He thought about where the breakthrough had actually come from. It hadn't been rare knowledge recalled at the right moment. It came from honoring dissonance: the visit count, the mismatch between records and recollection, the anger that never quite fit the physiology.

Once the problem representation crystallized, the diagnosis felt almost inevitable: subacute cognitive impairment and truncal ataxia in a surgically altered, nutritionally vulnerable patient with symmetric thalamic and mammillary body involvement.

But defining the problem was the true art. It meant resisting speed when the case looked easy. Treating repeated ED visits as abnormal vital signs. Allowing irritation to trigger curiosity instead of closure.

The diagnosis had been hiding inside a refill request.

And it almost stayed there.

Recap

- The key was not simply correcting hyperglycemia in someone missing insulin but asking why he was not taking insulin in the first place.
- Multiple emergency department visits are clinical data in their own right and warrant investigation.
- Identifying the real problem is the most important diagnostic step in clinical reasoning.

11

Reza had been practicing French for weeks.

He cleared his throat theatrically as they logged into the workstation. "*Bonjour, comment allez-vous?*" he greeted, careful and deliberate.

Rabih kept typing, shaking his head. "You say that like you're addressing a dignified stranger at a state dinner."

Reza tried again, brow furrowed in concentration. "*À tout aler… bisou bisou.*"

Rabih finally turned. "It's *à tout à l'heure.* And you can't say *bisou bisou* in the hospital."

Reza grinned. "Language is about confidence."

"It's also about grammar."

They were still laughing when the case dropped.

A 68-year-old man sat on the hospital bed inside an exam room, looked at them, and said, "Doc, I feel like I've aged ten years in the last three days."

Rabih pulled a stool to the bedside and sat. "Ten years?" he asked.

"That's right. I can't walk across the room without feeling like I'm going to pass out."

His wife stepped closer to the bed. “He’s never like this,” she said.

The patient repeated this, seeming irritated with himself. “If I stand up and try to walk, I get dizzy.”

It didn’t sound like the simple fatigue of a bad week. It was a loss of capacity. He felt fine lying down, but the moment he stood or walked, lightheadedness took over.

Pause and Reflect

What problem are we solving?

Exertional fatigue.

“Heart, lung, or blood,” Reza noted, thinking out loud with Rabih as they narrowed the field. Anemia. Arrhythmia. Low output state.

Before the differential settled, the monitor interrupted with a soft, repetitive beep—the kind heard a hundred times a day and usually ignored.

Heart rate: 27. Blood pressure: 102/70. Oxygen saturation normal.

The chief concern was exertional fatigue. The problem was bradycardia.

Management came first. Pads went on, cold adhesive touching the patient’s chest. IV access was secured. Atropine at the bedside. Blood pressure cycling every few minutes.

In unstable bradycardia, treatment must begin before the cause is fully known.

Figure 11.1

Symptomatic Bradycardia: Targeted and Empiric Treatment

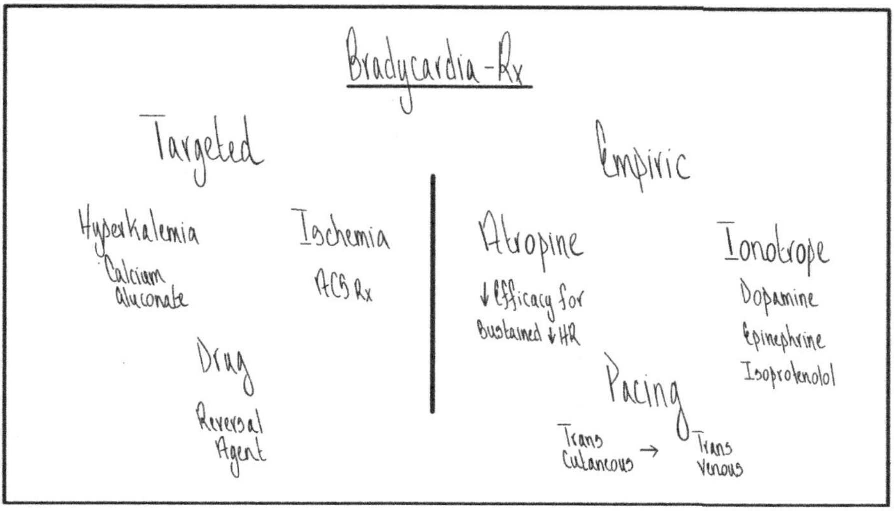

Unstable bradycardia requires immediate support that includes targeted treatment of specific conditions in addition to empiric treatment that helps all causes.

The EKG returned: *marked sinus bradycardia.* The sinus node was firing, just slowly.

Before treating a slow rhythm, decide whether the problem is extrinsic or intrinsic to the heart.

Figure 11.2

Acute Bradycardia: Extrinsic vs. Intrinsic Causes

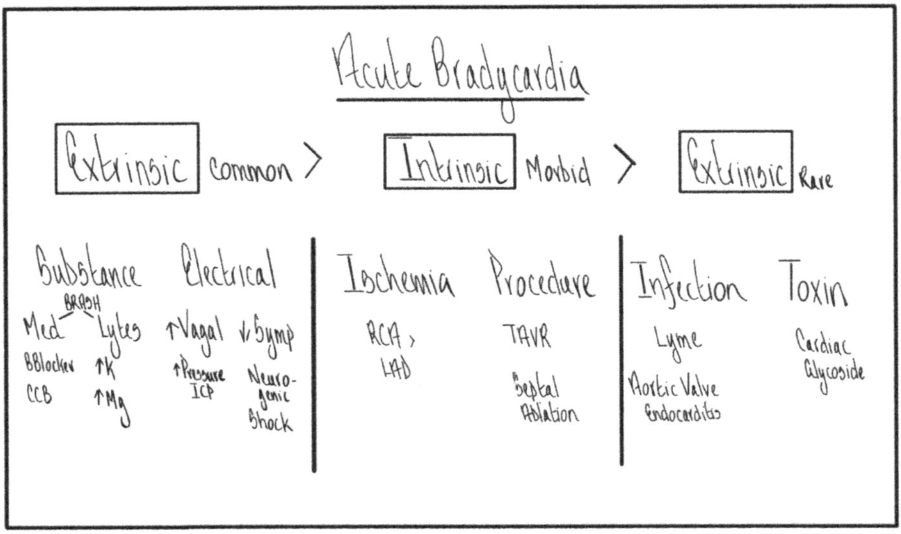

Extracardiac issues are the most common causes of bradycardia. Severe intrinsic diseases such as ischemia are less common but highly morbid.

What caused sinus bradycardia?

Drugs. Electrolytes. Ischemia. Endocrine. Vagal tone.

The patient took carvedilol, a small dose for hypertension and CKD. No recent changes. The mediset, a weekly pill organizer packed by his wife, had been filled in advance.

"Any chance you doubled up?"

He shook his head. His wife did too.

Labs returned within an hour: creatinine 1.6, baseline 1.3; potassium 4.8; magnesium and calcium normal; troponin negative; TSH normal. His heart rate sat in the low thirties. Nothing obvious declared itself.

Pause and Reflect

Could this be BRASH?

BRASH syndrome referred to the clinical cycle of bradycardia, renal failure, AV nodal blockade, shock, and hyperkalemia—a reinforcing loop in which renal dysfunction led to hyperkalemia, amplified AV nodal blockade, worsened bradycardia, lowered cardiac output, and further impaired renal perfusion.

The patient had CKD, was on a beta-blocker, and had a slightly elevated creatinine. The pieces almost fit. But the potassium was normal, and he was not hypotensive. The loop was not closed.

They next considered increased vagal tone. Acetylcholine slowed the sinus node, and on telemetry, heart rates commonly drifted into the forties during sleep without consequence. Athletes lived there comfortably at rest. That kind of slowing was expected, even healthy.

What was happening here was different: sustained bradycardia into the twenties in a symptomatic, awake patient. That was not typical vagal physiology.

While they were still working through the differential, a nurse checked a bladder scan.

"Post-void, nine hundred."

Nine hundred milliliters. His abdomen now appeared subtly distended—something easy to miss when alarms and pacing pads dominated the moment.

Pause and Reflect

Could urinary retention explain marked sinus bradycardia?

Retention was painful, which should result in a raised heart rate. Yet bladder distention stimulated pelvic afferents, and, in certain patients, that stretch could trigger an exaggerated vagal response. The wiring was not intuitive.

So a Foley was placed.

Before drainage, the patient's heart rate was 32.

1.2L of urine drained within minutes.

The monitor quickly climbed.

40.

52.

60.

67.

The alarm quieted. No atropine. No pacing. Just decompression, the simplest intervention undoing what had seemed so complex.

Later, the patient laughed, a sound of amusement and disbelief. "All that from not peeing?"

"When the bladder gets too full, it can send a signal that slows the heart," Rabih said, smiling as he sat down in a chair by the bedside. "Once we emptied it, the signal stopped, and everything reset."

The patient considered this. His wife shook her head slowly, making a noise that sounded like relief.

His heart wasn't failing. His conduction system was intact. His beta-blocker wasn't toxic.

His bladder was full.

Urology confirmed BPH, and alpha-blockade and finasteride were started with outpatient follow-up arranged.

In the hallway, Rabih lingered, collecting his thoughts. CKD, beta-blocker, mild creatinine bump, bradycardia. It had lined up neatly at first pass. He thought about how easy it would have been to stop there, to let the first coherent story win.

Inside the room, the pacer pads were still attached, unused. The monitor now showed a steady rate in the sixties.

Recap

- When a vague symptom obscures urgency, narrowing the frame step by step reveals the real problem, from fatigue to exertional fatigue to symptomatic bradycardia.
- Sinus bradycardia during sleep is normal, and it can be normal in a physically fit individual while awake. But, in a patient symptomatic from bradycardia, it is never normal and is often due to electrolyte derangements, drugs, or, less commonly, coronary ischemia or hypothyroidism.
- Frameworks like BRASH organize thinking, yet even when patterns appear to fit, the initiating trigger still must be found.

12

Rabih and Reza first met during their favorite hour of the day: morning report.

The conference room had filled slowly that morning, rows of metal chairs arranged in neat lines facing a single whiteboard. Coffee waited on a table in the back beside a box of bagels and tubs of cream cheese. The smell drifted through the room, mixing with the low murmur of residents greeting each other before the case began.

At the front stood the chief resident. Each year, the program selected one of its most outstanding graduating residents to stay on as chief. Part teacher, part organizer, and part referee, the chief resident guided the rhythm of the residency—and one of their most cherished roles was leading morning report.

Reza was two years ahead in residency, leaning back in his chair while the chief resident facilitated a case. The patient had gram-negative rod bacteremia after returning from rural Thailand, and the room buzzed with possibilities.

"What's the source?" the chief asked. "Urinary? Biliary? Gastrointestinal?"

A few answers from senior residents were offered.

Then a voice from the back said, calm but clear, "Could this be a breach in the intestines from *Strongyloides* hyperinfection?"

Reza's eyebrows lifted in quiet surprise, and he scanned the room, trying to find who had said it. A few other residents turned too. The suggestion was unusual but relevant to the case.

In the last row sat an intern he barely knew. He was wearing loose blue scrubs and a pair of worn Nike running shoes whose white had long ago faded to gray. He looked completely unconcerned with appearances, sitting slightly forward with his hands loosely folded, as if he had said the most ordinary thing in the world.

The chief rubbed his chin, looking thoughtful. "Say more."

The intern began to clarify his thought. "If strongyloidiasis disseminates, it can drag gut flora across the intestinal wall. Gram-negative bacteremia can be the clue."

Reza felt a flicker of admiration. Not because the answer was right or wrong, but because the reasoning was sound.

After the session, he walked over, weaving through the residents who were already filing out.

"That was a great thought," he said.

The intern looked up with the same easy composure he'd had when he spoke. "Thanks." He smiled, voice warm. "I'm Rabih. First week."

"I'm Reza. Want to grab coffee and think through the case?"

A decade later, they were side by side again in the emergency department.

Reza was scrolling through the chart as their patient said, "I haven't had a bowel movement in three days."

"We'll hydrate you, help you move your bowels, and get you comfortable."

Rabih tilted his head, watching the patient.

She was sixty-five, and she was perched at the edge of the bed, her shoulders drawn inward. Her heart rate read 110.

Rabih agreed that plain old constipation was likely, but something felt off.

She said her legs felt heavier than usual.

Rabih stepped closer to the bed. "Tell me what you mean by heavier."

The patient looked between them. "When I stand up," she said slowly, seeming to consider her answer, "it feels like I'm dragging them."

"Do they feel weak?" Rabih asked.

She shook her head. "Not weak. Just heavy."

Behind the curtain, the ED moved. Monitors warbled, a paramedic gave sign-out, and someone called for respiratory in room 2.

Reza looked at the monitor. "Her blood pressure's fine. She's afebrile."

Pause and Reflect

What are red flags for constipation?

Rabih paused, running through the mental checklist he taught residents. Red flags included abrupt onset, systemic symptoms, neurologic findings, or a lack of response to laxatives.

Constipation is common. Dangerous constipation announces itself through its pattern.

Figure 12.1

Constipation: Red Flags That Warrant Imaging or Further Evaluation

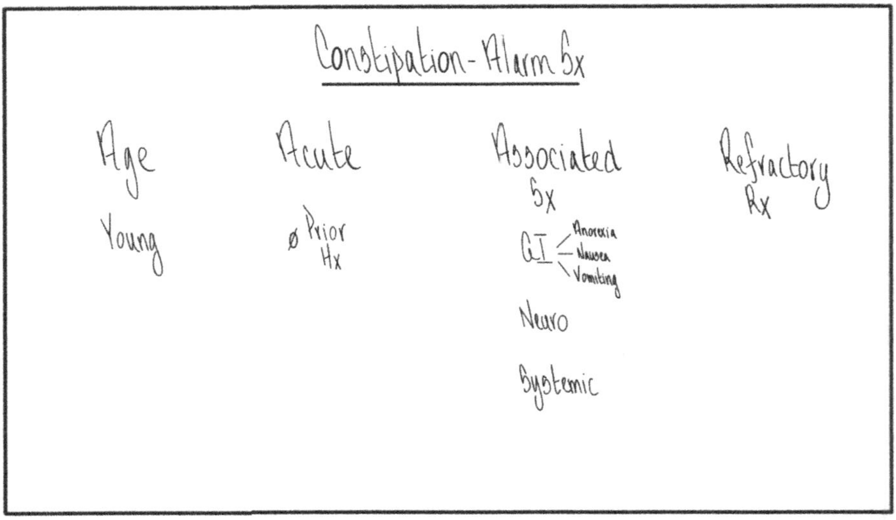

New or acute constipation, systemic symptoms, neurologic findings, anemia, urinary retention, or failure of standard therapy should prompt evaluation beyond symptomatic treatment.

They stepped into the hallway.

“New constipation in someone who has never had it,” Rabih said. “Persistent tachycardia. Subjective leg heaviness.”

Reza leaned against the wall. “Let’s hold both possibilities. Common things first, but we stay ready if the story changes.”

Thinking was free. Testing wasn’t.

Back in the room, Rabih slowed the history.

"No vomiting?"

"No."

"Belly pain?"

"Just pressure."

"Blood in the stool?"

"No."

"Back pain?"

The patient hesitated, her eyes shifting briefly to the ceiling. "Not really. I did have some pain near my left shoulder blade a couple of weeks ago. My chiropractor told me it was muscular."

Rabih looked at Reza. Something unspoken passed between them.

He asked about medications next.

"I started iron," she said. "My doctor said I'm anemic."

"When?"

"A week ago. Twice a day."

Reza tapped a pen against his badge, thinking. Starting iron made sense, and it was a common cause of constipation, especially at twice-daily dosing, but iron deficiency itself still needed a cause. Treatments were proximal explanations, not terminal ones.

Rabih studied the patient. "Any trouble peeing?"

She hesitated once more. "I'm going. Just not much."

With that in mind, they scanned her bladder. Five hundred twelve milliliters.

"Urinary retention," Rabih noted.

Reza studied the screen. "Could be incomplete emptying from constipation, but it definitely gets my attention."

A nurse who had been quietly adjusting the monitor spoke up without turning around. "I don't know if this helps," she said, "but she's been seen twice at urgent care for similar symptoms. She looked more uncomfortable walking in today."

Rabih faced her, intrigued. "That's important. Thank you."

He let her observation settle for a moment, then moved closer to the bedside to begin the neurologic exam. Strength full, reflexes symmetric, sensation intact. Gait cautious but steady.

Reza waited until the exam was finished before speaking. "Nothing neurologic is declaring itself yet. So we treat what we see and keep a low threshold to reassess."

They placed a Foley. Urine drained steadily into the bag, and her shoulders dropped slightly. They gave fluids next. Polyethylene glycol, senna, enema.

Hours passed. Rabih checked in on her twice. Her heart rate had fallen from 110 to 98 to 88.

"I feel lighter," she shared on his second visit, a faint smile tugging at the corners of her mouth.

The nurse returned to the bedside. "Large bowel movement," she reported.

The patient stood up, cautious at first, gripping the bedrail. But with each step, she seemed steadier. More sure of herself.

"Completely lighter?" Rabih asked.

"Not completely," she admitted. "But better."

Pause and Reflect

Should you get a CT scan of the abdomen?

Given her age, new symptoms, persistent tachycardia, recurrent presentations, and the sense that the pieces did not fully fit, they decided to get imaging before closing the loop.

A CT of the abdomen and pelvis showed mild stool burden without obstruction or mass, along with mild degenerative spinal disease. They discharged her with instructions, a bowel regimen, and strict return precautions.

At the workstation, Rabih reflected, "She mentioned scapular pain."

Reza rested his forearms on the desk. "Could be musculoskeletal. But let's document it so we can compare if she comes back."

Rabih agreed. Neither of them wanted to overreact, and neither wanted to ignore a signal that might declare itself later.

They cautiously assumed the lesson was over. It wasn't.

Two weeks later, the patient returned. Her heart rate was 112.

"My back," she reported. "It's not exactly pain. It's just there." She tapped below her left shoulder blade. "And my legs. They still feel heavy."

This time, neither Rabih nor Reza minimized it.

The neurologic exam was subtly different. Her ankle reflexes were softer, and her gait was more guarded. Nothing dramatic, but no longer clean.

In the hallway, Rabih stayed quiet, lost in thought.

Reza spoke up in his place. "I almost talked myself out of this again."

Labs showed persistent mild anemia. The rest of the CBC was normal, and the creatinine and calcium were normal.

Pause and Reflect

What would you do next?

They revisited the prior imaging with radiology, this time with a focus on the spine, given the back pain. The radiologist scrolled slowly through sagittal cuts.

"That's degenerative," he said at first. Then he paused. "Wait. Look there." A lytic lesion at L1. Additional scattered lesions.

Now the pattern cohered: new bowel dysfunction, urinary retention, subtle neurologic changes, scapular pain, and multiple visits over weeks.

Rabih leaned forward, silence stretching before he spoke. "When bowel and bladder slow together, one's usually driving the other," he said after a beat. "Constipation could explain the urinary retention."

"Or something's driving both," Reza said, eyes fixed on the screen. "Where does the cord end?"

"Around L1."

Reza looked up. "And what do the sacral segments of the spinal cord supply?"

"Bowel. Bladder."

When the bowel and bladder change together, localization comes before labeling.

Figure 12.2

Neurologic Dysfunction with Urinary Retention: Localization Framework

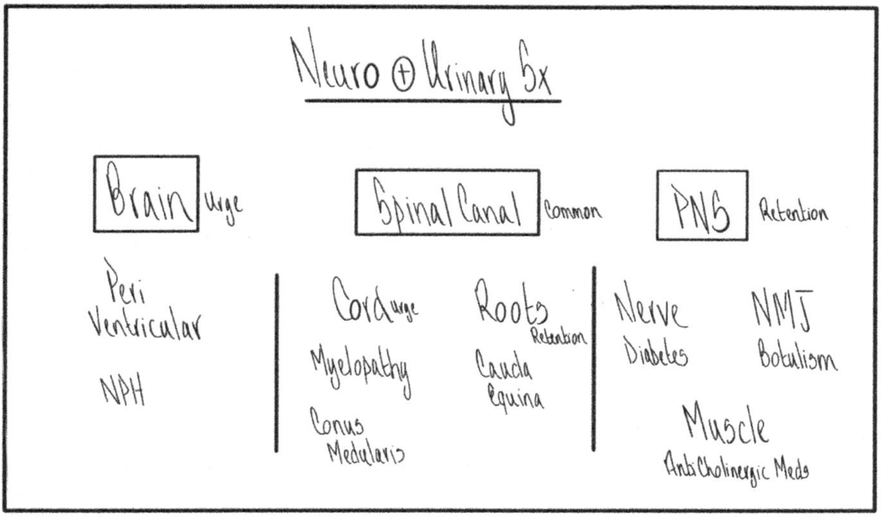

Concurrent bowel or bladder dysfunction with neurologic symptoms should prompt localization along the neuraxis—brain, spinal cord, nerve roots, peripheral nerves, neuromuscular junction, or medication effect.

A lesion at the level of the conus medullaris, around L1, did not need to announce itself with weakness. Autonomic dysfunction could come first—subtle signs that demanded careful attention.

Recognizing the urgency, steroids were started, and neurosurgery and oncology were called.

The protein studies returned with a large monoclonal spike and a markedly abnormal free light chain ratio.

Multiple myeloma.

In medical school, we were taught the CRAB mnemonic, which represented the four key features of the condition. Calcium elevation, renal insufficiency, anemia, and bone disease. But real presentations rarely unfolded in that order. Bone disease could appear early, while hypercalcemia often emerged later as the disease burden advanced.

They had primed their minds for the possibility of a rare cause of constipation, and when the symptoms evolved, they recognized the diagnosis early.

The patient underwent emergent surgery, was started on therapy for myeloma, and did well.

Recap

- Red flags for constipation include systemic symptoms, neurologic findings, abrupt onset, or presentation at a young age.
- Base rate matters, but hold less common causes in reserve so if the trajectory fails to improve as expected, you are ready to pivot without delay.
- Sometimes, reviewing prior tests is the most cost-effective path to a diagnosis.

13

A thirty-two-year-old woman sat hunched forward in a hospital bed, hands pressed against her temples, eyes clamped shut against the light.

"I've never had a headache like this," she said. "Not once."

Two days of excruciating pain, photophobia, nausea, and exhaustion.

"Doc, I can barely open my eyes."

When light itself becomes painful, localization begins at the eye and moves posteriorly.

Figure 13.1

Photophobia: Anatomic Localization Framework

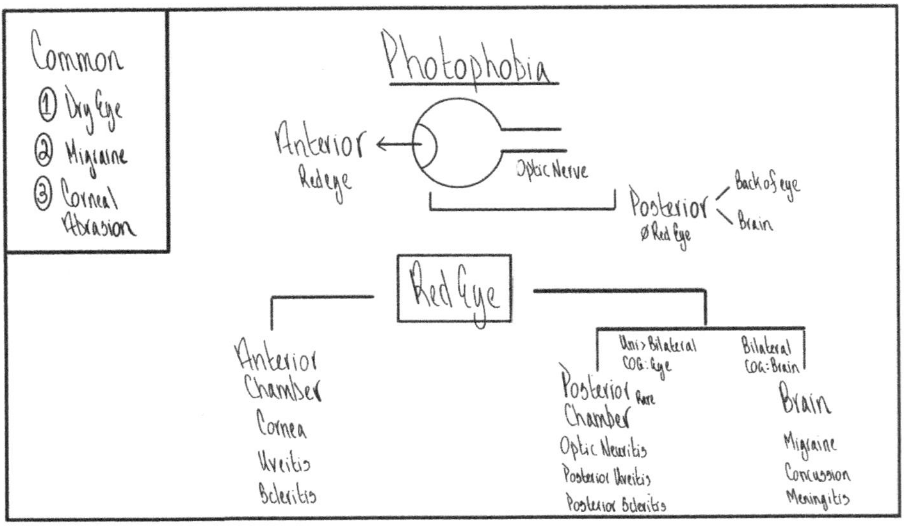

Photophobia with conjunctival injection suggests anterior ocular pathology such as corneal abrasion, uveitis, or scleritis. In the absence of red eye, posterior ocular or intracranial causes—including optic neuritis, migraine, or meningitis—should be considered.

The patient had no prior history of headaches and no records to review. She mentioned a splenectomy three years earlier for a benign lesion.

Rabih stood at the bedside. Reza dimmed the lights without a word.

The exam began immediately. Pupils equal and reactive, no conjunctival injection, extraocular movements intact, neck supple. No focal neurologic deficits.

Vitals appeared on the monitor. Afebrile. Hemodynamically stable.

They stepped into the hallway to discuss.

Before labeling a headache, look for red flags.

Figure 13.2

Headache: Clinical Features That Raise Concern for Secondary Causes

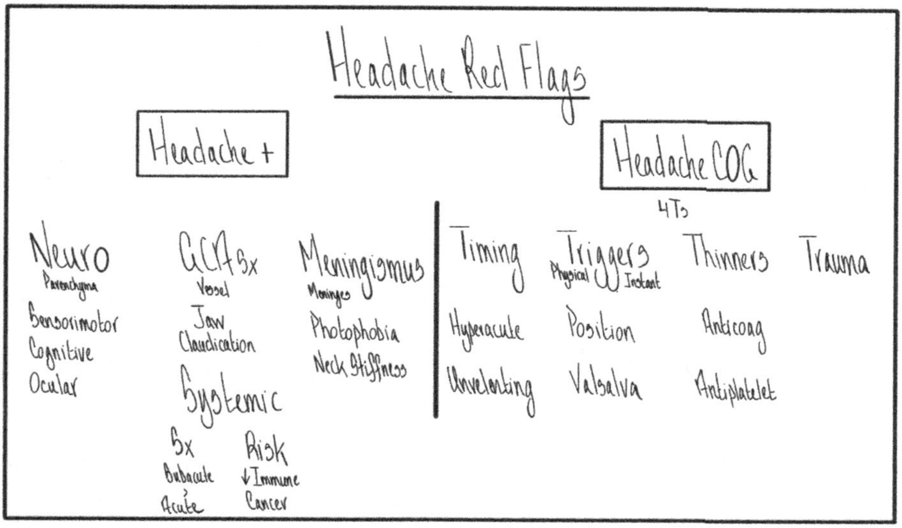

Headache accompanied by neurologic deficits, systemic illness, immunocompromise, hyperacute onset, positional triggers, trauma, or anticoagulation warrants urgent evaluation for secondary pathology.

Pause and Reflect

What is your approach to headache?

"Start outside the skull," Reza began. His voice stayed low, the way it often did when he was thinking aloud.

Rabih leaned against the wall, hallway lights humming faintly overhead. "Eyes. Sinuses. Teeth. Angle-closure glaucoma can masquerade. Sinus disease can mislead."

Reza hummed thoughtfully. "Then systemic. Infection, inflammation, metabolic stress. The head can complain when the culprit lives elsewhere."

"And only then do we move inward. Brain tissue. Vessels. Meninges."

Most headaches were primary. Migraine. Tension. The dangerous ones were the exception.

"History of splenectomy," Rabih noted.

Reza nodded. "Encapsulated organisms."

Photophobia without a spleen carried weight, even in the absence of fever.

Labs returned a few hours later. Rabih and Reza were in their workroom, the glow of the monitors casting shadows across their faces.

Normal white count. Normal chemistries. Each normal result nudged the probability downward, yet none erased their concern.

"If this is meningitis, delay matters," Rabih said, his voice low but firm.

Reza hummed thoughtfully, mentally weighing the risks. "If we're worried enough to tap for bacterial meningitis, should we get blood cultures and start antibiotics?"

Rabih ran a hand over his face, hesitation flickering in his eyes. "Maybe we should start with imaging."

A beat of silence passed between them. They sat there quietly, neither fully convinced.

Pause and Reflect

In a patient with a severe headache, photophobia, no prior history, and splenectomy, what is your next step?

Not entirely convinced this was meningitis, they reentered the room to reassess the patient. This time, they were accompanied by the resident.

The resident pulled a chair to the bedside, its legs scraping lightly against the tile. She sat, unhurried, and took a moment to look the patient over. Her gaze was piercing, as if she was scanning a chart come to life. Her first question seemed pointed. Directional. "Let me ask you something. How much coffee do you drink?"

The patient squinted, pain shadowing her features. "Six cups a day. At least."

"And your last one?"

"Two days ago. I stopped. My anxiety's been bad."

The timeline recalibrated. Two days. Abrupt cessation. Severe headache, photophobia, and nausea.

Caffeine withdrawal.

"Let's treat and observe."

They started fluids, antiemetics, and analgesia—keeping her comfortable while the withdrawal ran its course.

Two hours later, the patient sat upright, eyes open, light tolerable.

"It's fading," she said, relief creeping into her voice.

They deferred the lumbar puncture. They canceled the MRI. They discussed a gradual caffeine taper, explaining the risks of abrupt cessation.

When they called her days later, the headache had not returned.

Back at the workstation, Rabih caught Reza's attention. "We were ready to tap her and start antibiotics because of the spleen."

Reza exhaled, leaning back in his chair. "We were already halfway there."

They had respected the risk. But they had nearly let it outrun the data.

Rabih glanced toward the resident, who was finishing her note.

"We weren't that steady at her stage."

Reza shook his head, a small smile tugging at his lips. "The next generation is always the greatest generation."

Then he stood, stretching lightly. "I need coffee."

And after that encounter, he meant it.

Recap

- Bayesian reasoning is the discipline of recalibration. The absence of fever, leukocytosis, or neck stiffness does not individually rule out bacterial meningitis, but together, it shifts the probability sharply downward.

- Leadership in medicine is not about certainty. It is about creating the safest possible space for others to think out loud. Only then can the team see what any one clinician might miss.

14

The car rolled past red-brick buildings and row houses that seemed to lean toward the street, as if listening.

In the distance, a dome rose above the skyline.

Rabih broke the silence, hands resting loosely on the steering wheel. "You nervous?"

"A little," Reza admitted. "This place raised me."

"In five years?"

"In five years. My first faculty job."

Rabih smiled. "You used to walk by Osler every day."

Reza smiled back. "His portrait was on the ground floor, right by the elevator. I walked past it every single day. I finally took a selfie with him. I still wonder who wore the tie better."

"So, who did?"

Reza flashed a playful grin. "He did everything better. But I definitely made the tie look cooler."

He looked out the window for a moment. The dome now filled the windshield, pale against the morning sky.

Johns Hopkins Hospital.

Osler's hospital.

"My first day as faculty, I'm in the workroom. An intern presents and says, 'This is the Ashman phenomenon.' I freeze. I'm thinking, isn't Asherman gynecologic?" Reza said, shifting to look at Rabih. "But I nod and say, 'Classic Ashman.' I have no idea what I'm talking about. I go back to my office and Google it. Turns out Ashman beats reflect aberrant conduction seen in atrial fibrillation."

Rabih laughed, shaking his head fondly.

"And Rabih, it had absolutely nothing to do with the gynecologic system," Reza went on, grinning wryly at the memory.

Moments like that stayed with him. Over time, he finally learned how to say, "I don't know."

"This is where I'm surrounded by brilliant people who are committed to their patients," Reza continued. "The smartest people in the room are also the ones who care the most."

Rabih pulled into the parking lot. He gave one more encouraging smile before they exited the car and walked in.

The floors gleamed in that particular hospital way, clean but worn by decades of footsteps. They were visiting professors now, but for Reza, the building remained the place where he first learned how to build a team and how culture shaped the care patients received.

They joined rounds as the resident began presenting a patient.

Middle-aged, confused, transferred from a neighboring hospital. History notable for atrial fibrillation and moderate aortic stenosis. Liver enzymes in the thousands. INR elevated. No known history of chronic liver disease. No clear toxin exposure, no viral hepatitis. Blood pressure normal. Brain imaging unrevealing.

The room seemed to compress as the team looked at them, gazes heavy with expectation.

Pause and Reflect

What are your thoughts?

They paused on the term LFTs.

Reza looked around the room, taking in each set of attentive eyes. "First, let's clean up the language. AST and ALT aren't liver function tests. They reflect hepatocellular injury. For function, we want the INR, bilirubin, and albumin."

He continued, "And that distinction matters. Injury isn't the same as failure. Acute liver failure means loss of function—encephalopathy and coagulopathy—in someone without chronic disease. That changes the urgency. That can mean transplant."

A resident glanced back at the chart. "She has both. Confusion and an elevated INR."

Reza nodded. "Then by definition, this is failure."

Once injury and function are separated, acute liver disease becomes a localization problem: parenchyma, plumbing, or blood supply.

Figure 14.1

Acute liver disease: localize first

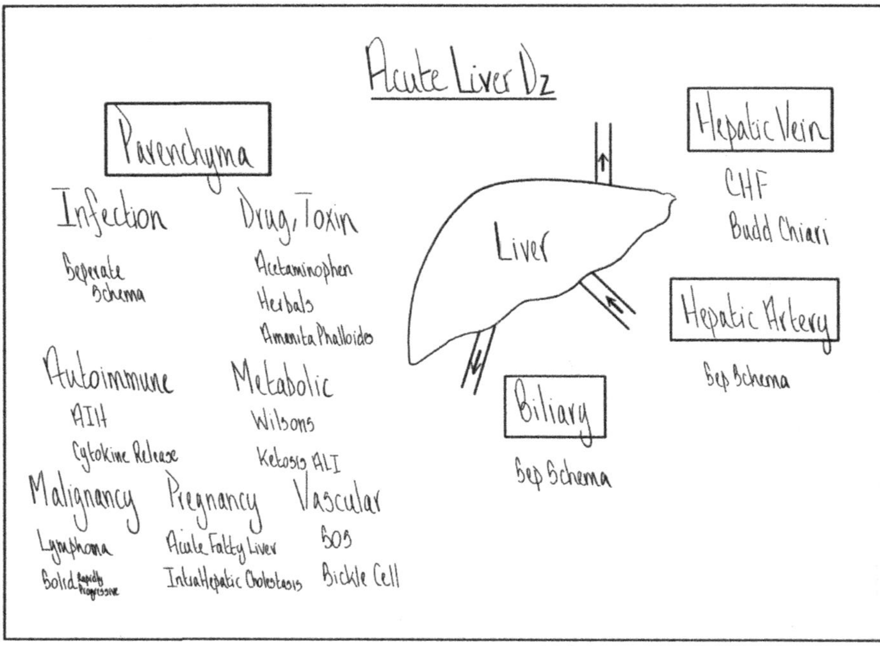

This framework separates parenchymal injury from biliary obstruction and vascular inflow/outflow failure because the compartment predicts the next tests and time-sensitive interventions.

Rabih folded his arms, leaning against the counter at the back of the room. "So, when you see numbers in the thousands, what comes to mind?"

A resident answered, "Ischemia. Toxins. Viral hepatitis."

"Good," Reza said. "Add acute biliary obstruction, though less common at this range. Now walk through them here."

"No toxin," another resident said. "Viral tests were negative. Imaging without obstruction."

Rabih asked, "So what's left?"

"Ischemia," someone said, voice sounding hesitant.

"But the blood pressure is normal," another resident added.

Over the next day, the patient's mental status cleared. Her liver enzymes fell.

Then something new appeared. Several toes became dusky. Cool. Blackening at the tips. Labs showed disordered clotting, with concern for disseminated intravascular coagulation.

Now there were two dots.

Transient acute liver failure.

A clotting disorder with peripheral gangrene.

Two dots. No line between them.

The team returned to the workroom, the hum of computers and low chatter filling the air.

A senior resident spoke up.

"Let's go back to the first hour."

He pulled up the outside records and reviewed the timeline again. And then he saw it: severe hypotension at the neighboring hospital.

Ischemic hepatitis is the diagnosis that gets missed when we anchor on the vitals in front of us instead of the hemodynamics that came before.

Figure 14.2

Ischemic hepatitis: pattern + physiology

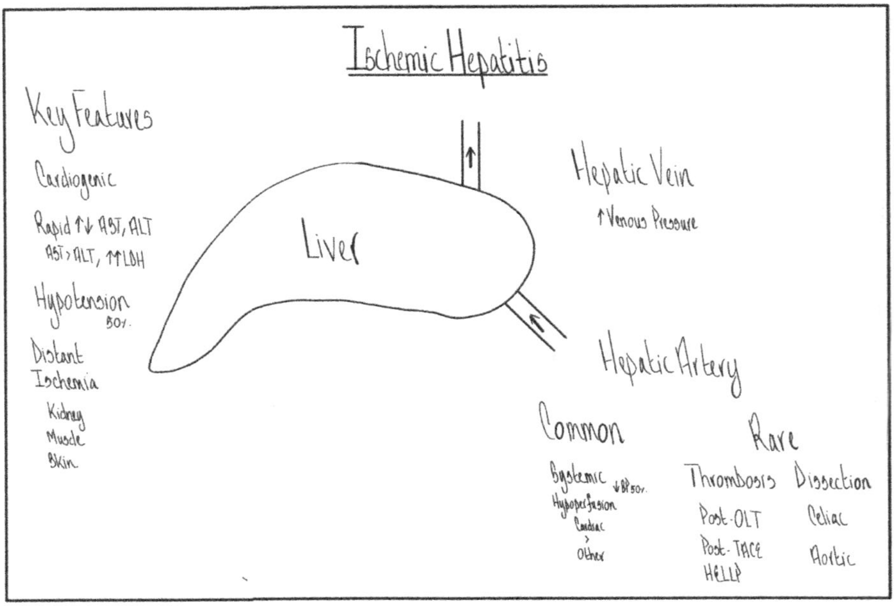

A sudden AST/ALT surge with a high LDH and rapid improvement after perfusion returns points to ischemia, even when hypotension is no longer present.

"Wow," Rabih said, his tone emphatic, "Normal now doesn't mean it was normal before."

Low volume, rapid atrial fibrillation, impaired filling across a stenotic valve. The liver became ischemic—shock liver. Transient, if reversed quickly.

Fluids were given, and the blood pressure was restored. The liver recovered.

Dot one.

But what about the toes?

Pause and Reflect

What explains the digital gangrene?

Reza looked at the senior resident, not knowing the answer himself and crowdsourcing. "How can someone clot and have an elevated INR at the same time?"

The resident thought for a moment. "Because the liver makes both procoagulant and anticoagulant proteins. Synthesis stops," he continued, "but not everything disappears at the same speed."

Reza, already impressed, asked, "Which falls first?"

"The anticoagulant factors," the resident responded. "So, for a brief window, the procoagulant factors persist without their balance."

Rabih added, "And the system tilts."

"Toward thrombosis," the resident finished.

Micro-clots formed within days. Digits darkened. Dot two. Transient hypotension caused ischemic hepatitis, and the recovery left behind a dangerous imbalance in coagulation that played out in the periphery.

The patient improved, but ultimately, the necrotic digits required amputation.

The resident explained the chain of events to the patient and her family. He didn't stop when the liver enzymes improved; he kept asking why. There was sadness in the room, but there was also clarity.

Recap

- When AST and ALT rise into the thousands, distinguishing severe hepatocellular injury from true liver failure is critical because failure changes urgency, disposition, and the possibility of transplant.

- Psychological safety is not about comfort; it is about creating a culture where uncertainty can be voiced so better thinking can occur.

- Never stop asking why, because deeper understanding can change management and bring clarity to patients and families.

15

Night shift.

Reza was in his office watching YouTube golf.

The volume was low but audible. The instructor's voice sounded calm, confident, certain. *"Shift your weight before the downswing. Let the club fall into the slot."*

On the screen, a perfect drive traced a slow white arc against a blue sky. Frame by frame, the hips rotated, the wrists hinged, and the clubface squared. Reza stood up from his chair and mimicked the motion, a half swing in the narrow space between desk and door. Pause at the top, slow rotation. He checked his reflection in the dark window.

His pager interrupted the illusion of improvement.

"Blood pressure 83 over 48."

Reza called back.

"Is she symptomatic?" he asked.

"No," the nurse said. "She's talking. Says she feels fine."

Reza and Rabih both knew the patient well; they had been caring for her for weeks. She was in her seventies, lived on the edge of perfusion even on good days, and carried an ejection fraction of 20%. Schizophrenia.

Probate conservator. A month in the hospital already.

He opened the chart while still on the phone. A similar page three nights ago. Documented assessment: *Baseline asymptomatic hypotension.*

He scrolled further back. For weeks, her systolic blood pressure had drifted between the high 80s and low 90s. The pattern offered some reassurance, but still, he knew he could not manage hypotension from a chair.

The patient was awake and conversational when Reza entered the room. Her other vitals were normal. No chest pain, no lightheadedness. She told him she felt about the same. Her neck veins were distended, and her legs were edematous. Her skin was warm.

He rechecked the blood pressure. Ninety-six over sixty. Higher than the page. He thanked the nurse, documented the assessment, and returned to his office. The golf video was still paused mid-swing.

The weekend came, and now Rabih was covering. He was in the workroom, eyes mindlessly flicking over an article, when his pager buzzed against his hip. He glanced at the screen.

"Systolic 76."

He recognized the name and hesitated, fingers hovering over the pager. The number was close to the patient's baseline.

Still, he called back. The nurse answered, and it was something in her voice, more than anything she said, that gave him pause. He told her he'd come by.

The patient was awake when he arrived, propped up in the bed and answering the nurse's questions in full sentences. Rabih moved to the bedside, smiling at the patient while his eyes scanned her. Her lower extremity edema and jugular venous distention were still present, but they looked largely unchanged. Her oxygen saturation was normal.

The nurse rechecked the blood pressure in the other arm, yielding a reading in the mid-80s, near the patient's baseline.

Rabih left feeling settled. He walked back to the workroom, flopped into his chair, and clicked on a monitor. A few minutes of charting passed.

Then the nurse called again.

"She gets fatigued with small movements," she said. "Just walking to the bathroom wipes her out."

That was new.

The nurse continued. She'd obtained an EKG that looked abnormal. She asked Rabih to come take a look.

He studied it. Progressive PR lengthening and dropped beats. It looked like Mobitz type I, though he wasn't fully confident.

He pulled out his phone and snapped a picture, sending it to Reza with a caption reading *"??"* Reza texted back a moment later, offering the same conclusion. Mobitz I. Still, an internal hesitation, or perhaps a need to be certain, was enough to escalate his concern and send the EKG to the cardiology attending.

He was still waiting to hear back when the nurse paged once more. *"No urine output since this morning."*

Pause and Commit

What is your next diagnostic and therapeutic move for this patient's hypotension?

When arterial pressure falls, the next question is whether venous pressure is low or elevated.

Figure 15.1

Hypotension: Arterial Pressure and Venous Pressure

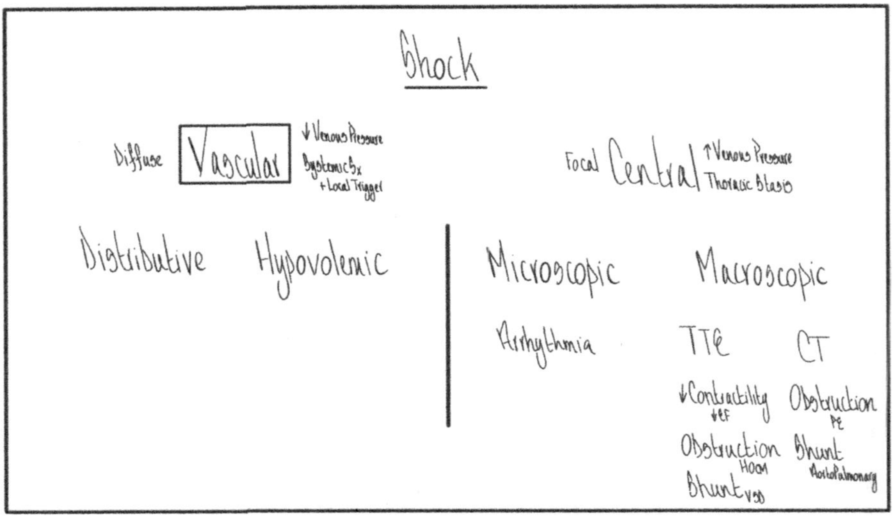

Hypotension alone is incomplete information. The number tells you that forward flow is low, but it does not tell you why. The first branch point is venous pressure.

Rabih framed the problem as arterial hypotension with venous hypertension, given the JVD and lower extremity edema in the context of a known low EF.

He considered cardiogenic shock but, upon further examination, found her extremities warm.

He ordered labs—BMP, CBC, LFTs, lactate—along with a chest X-ray and requested strict monitoring of her intake and output. Review of her medications and prior notes confirmed that the only drugs she was taking were furosemide and, intermittently, metoprolol.

But the patient rejected the labs and imaging.

Rabih and the nurse moved to the hallway to discuss.

"I'm glad you were worried," he said.

"I just feel like something's off," the nurse replied. "Her pressure alone doesn't scare me. But the fatigue, the urine output… that changes the picture."

Rabih chewed on his lower lip. "If she's drifting toward cardiogenic shock, we need to know. And if she's stable, that matters too. We need these labs."

"I'll try again," the nurse said, disappearing into the room.

Rabih moved to the workstation, ordering telemetry and trying to reach the probate conservator.

Around that time, the cardiology attending texted him back.

"Not Mobitz I."

Rabih watched the typing bubble appear, disappear, and appear again. He stared at the screen, waiting.

"Atrial flutter with variable block. With her low EF, she depends on atrial kick. That's likely driving the hypotension."

Rabih read it twice. Then he remembered: the nurse had mentioned a flicker in the patient's neck veins, just before the EKG was obtained. He hadn't known what to make of it at the time. Now it made sense. It was the flutter waves.

It helps to step back and define what atrioventricular block represents: a problem of communication between atrium and ventricle.

Figure 15.2

Atrioventricular Block: Integrity of Conduction

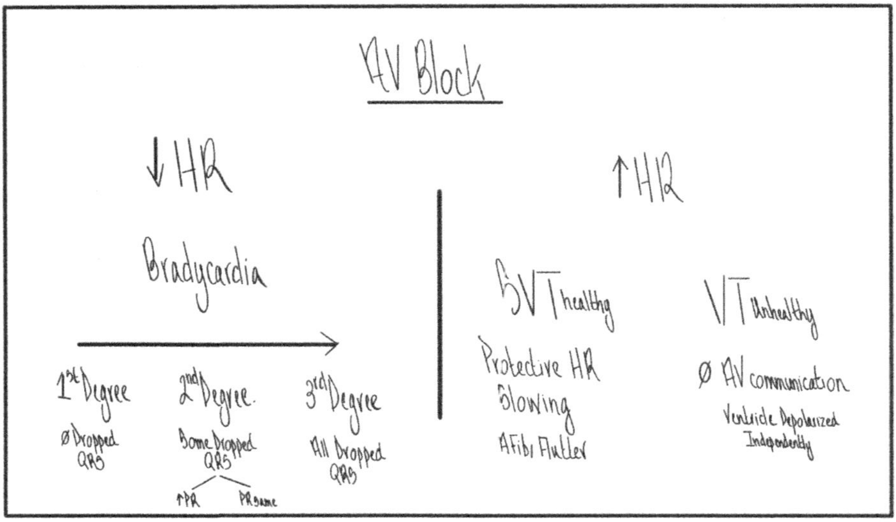

AV block is a healthy physiologic phenomenon in patients with a supraventricular tachycardia protecting the ventricle from excessive beating. In other scenarios, it is a marker of a potentially serious underlying cause.

Pause and Commit

Now that you know the correct interpretation of the EKG, how does it change your management?

The patient had now refused labs three times.

The nurse pulled a chair to the bedside and sat down, schooling her expression into something gentle.

"Can you tell me what worries you about the blood draw?" she asked, her voice a soothing hum.

"I'm afraid of needles," the patient answered. "I hate them."

"That makes sense," the nurse affirmed. She didn't reach for a counter-argument; she didn't pivot or patronize. She just let the answer be what it was. "Is it the pain? Or something else?"

The patient seemed to think for a moment, blinking slowly at the nurse. "The whole thing, I think. The waiting, and then it happens, and I—" she broke off for a moment. Then concluded in a quiet tone, "I just hate it."

"I understand," the nurse said. "A lot of people feel that way."

A few seconds passed. The monitor beeped quietly in the corner, and somewhere down the hall, a door clicked shut.

"What would make it easier?" the nurse asked, shifting closer.

The patient stayed silent for a beat, as if the question were foreign. As if no one had thought to ask her before. "If you stay with me while they do it," she finally said. "Don't leave."

"I won't," the nurse said. "I'll be right here."

When phlebotomy returned, the nurse stood at the bedside. She talked softly about nothing in particular, one hand resting on the patient's shoulder. The patient looked at the ceiling. Her jaw was tight, but she held still.

The blood was drawn.

Rabih signed out to Reza a little while later and headed home. He had just settled on his sofa, açai bowl in hand, Champions League highlights on the TV, when his phone buzzed on the cushion beside him.

"You won't believe this. Her hemoglobin came back at 6. It was 10 a month ago. Iron levels are low. She's significantly iron deficient."

Rabih set the açai down. *"No way,"* he typed back. *"The nurse said she looked pale before we even sent the labs."*

He sat with that for a moment as Reza texted him the other results. Lactate normal, renal function slightly worsened.

He leaned back and looked at the ceiling, the pieces clicking into place before him. The patient likely had slow blood loss and developed iron deficiency anemia. In a heart with an ejection fraction of 20%, she depended on atrial contraction to fill a weak ventricle. The anemia likely triggered atrial flutter, and without that atrial kick, her stroke volume dropped. In that setting, hypotension followed. The combination of anemia and loss of atrial contribution explained her exertional intolerance.

Later, in a meeting with the patient and her conservator, the decision was made to transition her to hospice. Further pokes and tests were no longer consistent with her values.

But now, still sprawled on the sofa, Rabih called Reza.

"The nurse knew," he said as soon as the call connected.

"She did."

"The pressure was low for weeks. We called it baseline. She didn't; she saw the trajectory. Not just the number we kept calling stable." Rabih spoke quickly, his thoughts a blur of the day, the case, and the patient he almost let slip through the cracks. "She noticed the fatigue, the urine, the flicker in the neck, the pallor. We needed labs and an EKG to name it. She saw it at the bedside."

"That's the difference," Reza answered, his voice slower, as if working it out in real time. "They're there all day. They catch the subtle shifts before we do."

"And we almost didn't see it at all."

Recap

- When you are not confident in the interpretation of a piece of data, ask for help; here, reframing the EKG led to the discovery of severe iron deficiency anemia and the true driver of the atrial arrhythmia.

- In hypotension, always ask what the venous pressure is; elevated venous pressure should shift your thinking toward cardiogenic shock and demand further investigation.

- Bedside nurses see trajectory before physicians do, and listening to their specific observations is not courtesy—it is clinical excellence.

16

The page: *"Lower extremity edema."*

It was a busy admitting day. Rabih and Reza were on the inpatient service, evaluating patients in the emergency department. The waiting room was full, a whirlwind of noise and illness.

The page described a fifty-eight-year-old man. Out of care for years, up twenty pounds in the last four months. The CT report was already in the chart, confidently describing cirrhotic morphology.

They stepped into the room and introduced themselves. The patient was sitting upright on the gurney, legs hanging off the side. His socks were off, revealing visibly swollen feet that ballooned at the edges. His face looked tired, but he was alert, tracking every word.

Rabih started the way he always did, gentle and direct. "Tell us what you've noticed."

"My legs," the patient answered, patting his shins. "They're huge. And I'm getting heavier. I don't eat like that."

Reza shifted slightly toward Rabih. The reflex was already there. The organ frame. Heart, liver, kidney. Venous stasis.

Rabih kept his voice patient-facing. "We're going to examine you, and we'll think out loud as we go. If anything doesn't make sense, stop us."

The patient shrugged. "Go ahead."

His BP was normal. Not hypotensive, not hypertensive. Oxygen saturation intact. No crackles. JVP unimpressive. A few spider angiomata on the chest. No jaundice, no caput.

Reza knelt, pressing a thumb into the shin, and watched the indentation linger. Bilateral pitting edema, obvious. But as he reached for the next step in the usual script, something felt off.

Rabih lifted the patient's forearm and pressed along the wrist. The skin gave the same slow, soft pit.

"Your arms are swollen too," Rabih noted, glancing at a few tattoos dotting the forearm as he spoke.

The patient blinked. "Yeah. I had to take my watch off. And my ring too. A few weeks ago."

A dent appeared on the lateral thigh as Reza moved his hand there and pressed down.

Rabih studied the patient's face, quietly observant. There was a faint puffiness around the eyes that became apparent once he noticed it. He kept his tone calm. "You've also got some swelling around your eyes, and your belly looks more full."

The patient exhaled, seeming relieved that someone was naming what he'd been feeling. "I thought I was just getting fat."

Reza thought about the CT report for a moment. Cirrhotic morphology. A tempting answer, a confident report. But the body in front of him was telling a wider story.

So he diverted his attention back to the patient. "Before we go further, has anyone ever told you that you have liver disease or cirrhosis?"

The patient shook his head. "No."

"Your imaging describes a liver that looks stiff," Reza continued, "but imaging alone doesn't make that diagnosis. We'll work that up properly. What's important right now is that this degree of swelling is more than we'd expect the liver to explain by itself, so we need to look broadly at other causes."

Rabih added, "This is anasarca."

The patient repeated the word like he was trying it on. "An...asarca."

"It just means generalized swelling," Rabih said. "And it changes what we have to consider."

Pause and Commit

This is not just lower extremity edema. It is anasarca. How does that change your differential diagnosis?

The first step is to separate typical causes of edema from processes that produce true anasarca.

Figure 16.1

Anasarca

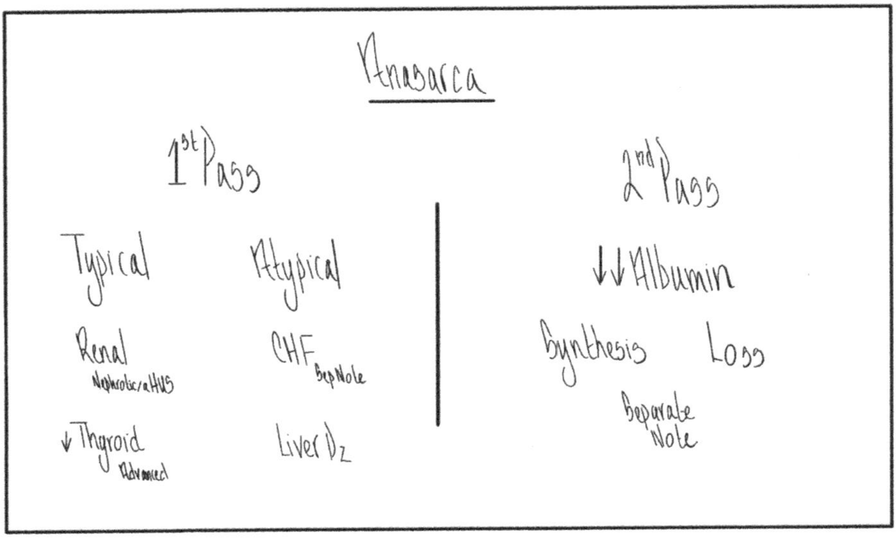

Anasarca represents generalized edema involving multiple body compartments. Renal and thyroid diseases are the most common causes in all comers.

Reza kept his eyes on the patient, careful not to turn the bedside into a lecture that left him behind. "It makes us think about conditions that lower the protein in the blood, like kidney disease that spills protein into the urine. It also makes us think about thyroid disease and about problems where fluid leaks out of the blood vessels."

Rabih followed the direction of Reza's reasoning. Not chronic kidney disease. Nephrotic syndrome.

Rabih added, "We'll still evaluate the liver, especially because the CT suggested it. But we don't want to anchor on one explanation when your swelling is this widespread."

The patient shifted slightly on the gurney. "So what happens next?"

"We'll start with a focused set of labs and urine tests," Reza answered.

Rabih offered a small smile. "We'll keep you in the loop."

"This is swelling turned system-wide," Rabih remarked as they stepped just outside the curtain.

"And hypothyroidism deserves real space," Reza said. "Not as an afterthought."

Rabih looked back toward the bed. "And it keeps us honest about the CT. Cirrhosis can be real, but generalized edema broadens the differential."

"And that difference matters because it dictates what we consider next."

Back in the workroom, the labs began to populate.

Creatinine normal. Albumin 1.8.

When the albumin is this low, the question becomes whether the body is making less of it or losing it somewhere.

Figure 16.2

Approaching Hypoalbuminemia

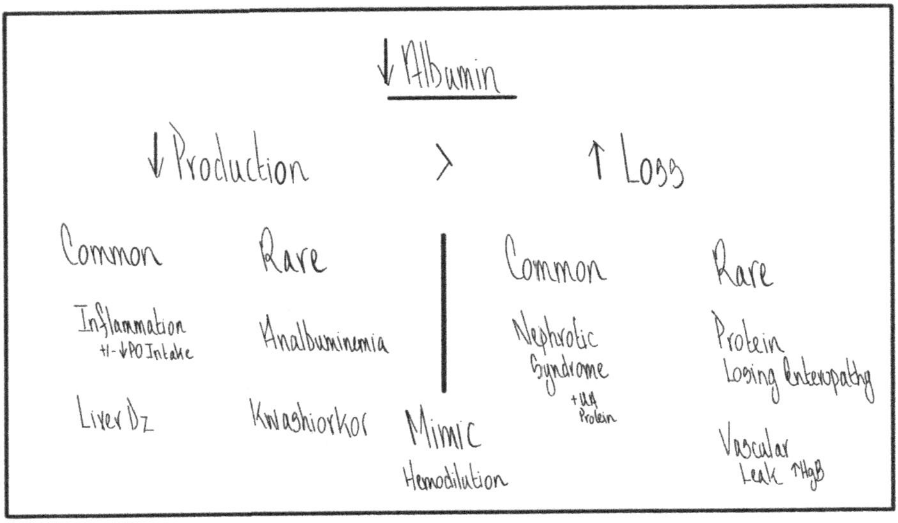

Severe hypoalbuminemia results from either reduced production or increased loss.

Rabih pulled his chair closer to Reza's, both of them now settled in the workroom. "INR?"

"Normal."

"Bilirubin?"

"Also normal. And the platelets are 165," Reza noted. "If this were advanced cirrhosis driving this degree of edema, why is albumin the only synthetic marker down?"

Rabih thought for a moment. “Severely low albumin has a short differential. Decreased production from liver dysfunction. Reduced synthesis in systemic inflammation. Or loss—usually kidney, less often gut.”

Reza scrolled through more lab values. “No evidence of a systemic inflammatory illness. And the albumin feels out of proportion to the rest of the liver profile.”

“Loss moves up,” Rabih said. “Kidney first. Gut is rarer, and he doesn’t have GI symptoms.”

The BNP returned low. Mild AST and ALT elevation. Urine tox screen with methamphetamine.

Then the urinalysis populated.

Reza straightened. “There’s protein in the urine. 100+. And a few red cells.” He scrolled back up, then down again. “Severely low albumin with proteinuria isn’t incidental. We need a urine protein to creatinine ratio.”

The spot protein to creatinine ratio returned that night: 3.27.

A day later, the 24-hour urine confirmed it. Twelve grams of proteinuria.

Rabih, in the workroom again, exhaled slowly. “Okay. Triad is there.”

“Nephrotic-range proteinuria,” Reza said.

“Hypoalbuminemia.”

“Edema.”

This was nephrotic syndrome.

Pause and Reflect

How do you explain the normal blood pressure in nephrotic syndrome?

Rabih swiveled toward Reza. "The blood pressure being normal doesn't reassure me. Cirrhosis tends to vasodilate. Nephrotic states can expand volume. Two forces in opposite directions can look normal."

"Normal doesn't mean neutral," Reza said, nodding.

Now the question had shifted.

"Why nephrotic?" Reza asked.

Pause and Reflect

What could explain both the nephrotic syndrome and radiographic cirrhosis?

Rabih counted on his fingers as he talked through his approach to nephrotic syndrome. "Primary patterns include membranous, FSGS, minimal change. But secondary causes matter more here."

Reza added, "Tattoos. Methamphetamine on the urine screen. Out of care for years."

"One process that can hit both liver and kidney?"

The hepatitis panel returned within a couple of hours.

Reza read aloud. "Hepatitis C antibody positive. Viral load 4.4 million."

"The liver disease is real," he concluded. "But it's not carrying the whole story."

Complement levels drifted low. Rheumatoid factor negative.

Reza pointed at the urinalysis again. "Red cells persist. That's nephritic flavor layered onto nephrotic."

Pause and Reflect

What is the differential diagnosis when there is an overlap of nephrotic and nephritic syndrome?

Rabih leaned back. "Lupus. IgA. MPGN."

"In a patient with hepatitis C," Reza said, "MPGN moves forward."

A kidney biopsy revealed membranoproliferative glomerulonephritis.

The cryoglobulin screen returned positive. Cryocrit 1 percent.

The arc had now closed. Hepatitis C was driving immune-complex deposition in the kidney. Nephrotic syndrome was driving the edema. Cirrhosis was present, likely from the same virus, but it was not the primary engine of the fluid.

The patient became oliguric. Loop diuretics alone did little. Nephrology recommended intravenous albumin followed by a diuretic, and he diuresed briskly. The creatinine drifted down; edema softened.

Later, they sat at the workstation, the ED still loud around them. The waiting room hadn't emptied.

"We almost let a radiographic label outrank a lab inconsistency," Reza said, his voice contemplative.

"We almost treated albumin as synonymous with liver," Rabih added. "And almost forgot to quantify protein loss."

The realization lingered: anasarca did not narrow the differential; it broadened and prioritized it.

Recap

- Defining the correct problem is the only reliable path to a timely and accurate diagnosis, and distinguishing leg edema from anasarca fundamentally reshapes the differential.
- Attend to the degree of abnormality rather than labeling values as simply high or low; a severely low albumin out of proportion to the rest of the liver profile demands a broader explanation.
- Any patient with anasarca deserves a spot urine protein to creatinine ratio early in the evaluation.

17

They met up outside Reza's favorite restaurant, Chipotle. He ordered the same thing he always did, a burrito with double chicken, no beans, extra corn, sour cream, cheese, and mild salsa, and they sat down on a bench with their burritos wrapped in foil. The smell of grilled chicken and warm tortillas drifted through the air. Cars idled nearby. Someone laughed behind them. It felt comfortingly ordinary.

Rabih leaned back and studied Reza's face longer than usual.

"You look tired," he said.

"Overnight shift," Reza answered too quickly, the words sounding false on his tongue.

Rabih nodded, but his eyes held a beat too long.

After a decade of friendship, small things gave them away. Cadence shifts. Posture changes. Eyes holding or avoiding contact in ways they never used to. Rabih noticed Reza's unusual demeanor before he said another word.

"Reza," he said softly. "What's going on?"

Reza looked down at the burrito in his hands. The foil crinkled as his grip tightened around it.

"I was going to tell you later," he said. "Maybe even talk about it on the podcast." His voice caught. "It's my dad."

Rabih didn't interrupt. His gaze stayed on Reza, unwavering.

"His PSA was slightly elevated. They ordered a prostate MRI. The prostate looked fine." Reza swallowed. "But they found retroperitoneal lymphadenopathy."

A CT of the abdomen and pelvis confirmed the retroperitoneal nodes and showed inguinal lymphadenopathy too, left greater than right.

Rabih went quiet, his expression shifting into something familiar. Reza saw the slight narrowing of his focus, the way he looked into the distance when his mind started organizing possibilities. He didn't say anything yet, but Reza knew he was building a differential.

Pause and Reflect

What is your approach to lymphadenopathy? Does retroperitoneal location prioritize anything?

When lymphadenopathy is diffuse and involves deep nodal stations, the differential diagnosis shifts toward systemic processes rather than localized infection.

Figure 17.1

Disseminated Lymphadenopathy

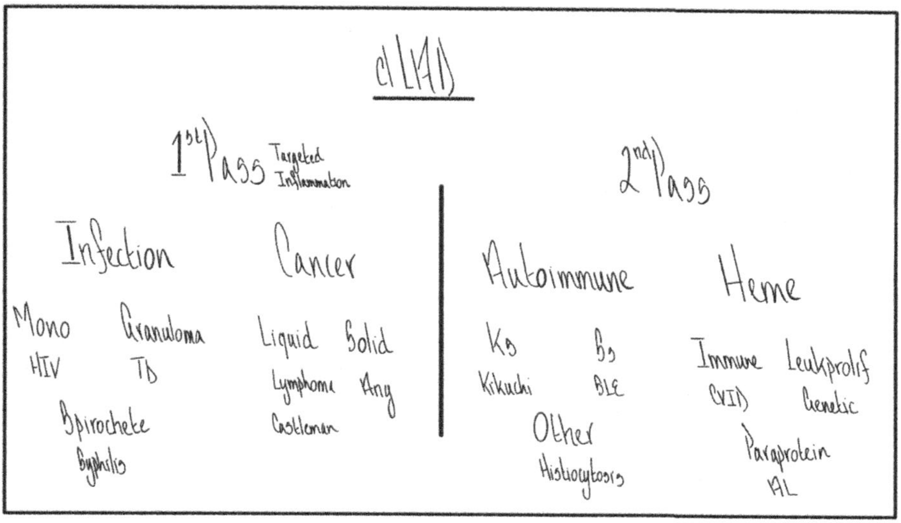

Disseminated lymphadenopathy most often reflects systemic disease. Infections and cancers are the leading causes.

Retroperitoneal nodes. Reza felt his mind slipping into familiar territory. The location alone shifted the weight of the differential. His first instinct was malignancy. The question became what kind: a primary lymphoid process or a metastatic solid tumor.

If it was metastatic, the next question was about its origin. He started tracing drainage patterns in his head. Rectal cancer. Prostate cancer. Melanoma from the leg. Testicular cancer. But the details didn't line up. His father's colonoscopy a year earlier was normal. No change in bowel habits. No bleeding, no skin lesions on the legs. No palpable testicular mass. The prostate MRI was reassuring, and the CT showed no obvious primary tumor.

Reza tried to make metastasis fit anyway, but it kept sliding backward.

Infection trailed behind. Tuberculosis had crossed his mind; his father was born in Iran. But there were no fevers, no inflammatory markers, no constitutional symptoms.

Autoimmune diseases such as IgG4-related disease or sarcoidosis could cause retroperitoneal lymphadenopathy, but they rarely presented in isolation.

Reza kept coming back to the same place. Deep abdominal lymphadenopathy without an obvious inflammatory trigger made lymphoma hard to ignore.

He paused, letting the thought settle in his chest. The patient he had been thinking about so clinically was his father, the man who taught him how to ride a bike, work through the Pythagorean theorem, and calculate the velocity of a moving object.

"I called the radiologist," Reza said, breaking the silence. One hand was absently tracing the wood of the bench.

"After hours?" Rabih asked.

"Yes. I know the reading room number." Reza hesitated before going on. "I felt bad using that access. But this is my dad."

Rabih didn't judge. A tiny nod, almost imperceptible, told Reza he understood.

"Some of the inguinal nodes are clustered around major vessels," Reza continued, biting his lower lip as he spoke. "The radiologist recommended biopsy."

They both knew what that meant.

In these situations, most roads led to tissue. But before tissue, they slowed down.

Pause and Reflect

What causes of lymphadenopathy can be diagnosed on blood tests alone?

A small group of conditions can produce lymphadenopathy yet still be diagnosed through blood testing alone.

Figure 17.2

Lymphadenopathy Diagnosable Without Biopsy

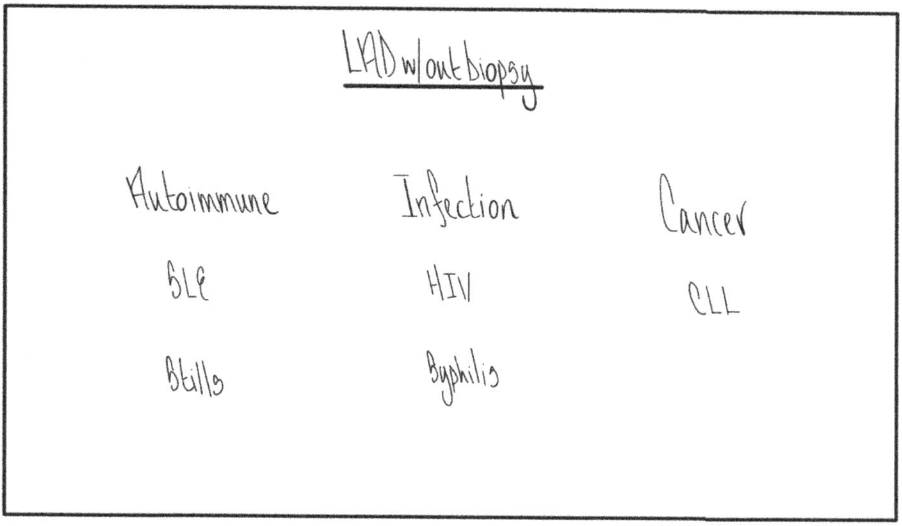

Although tissue diagnosis is often required for lymphadenopathy, several important causes can be diagnosed through blood testing.

Reza had already considered the least invasive possibilities. HIV, EBV, CMV. Syphilis. Tuberculosis. Autoimmune diseases such as lupus or Sjögren's.

Serology. PCR. Because the answer might already be circulating in the blood.

But his father's labs were normal.

"How bad can this be?" Reza asked, eyes searching out Rabih's. "He feels completely fine." He was asking questions he knew the answer to. When the patient was your father, clarity slipped.

Rabih squinted toward the street, as if searching beyond the cars passing by.

"There's a disconnect," he said. "Clinical and radiographic. But the nodes are real. Something's driving them."

That thought lingered between them, uncomfortable and unresolved. Neither moved to rise, instead remaining on the bench, holding burritos that had gone cold.

A biopsy was scheduled for two weeks later.

Rabih called that same evening, not long after the appointment had been set. "I can't stop thinking about it," he said.

He didn't mean the biopsy. He meant all of it: the weight of watching a parent move through something that you, even being a doctor, could not fix. He spoke about his own father, about the Parkinson's, about watching decline slowly unfold. A tremor here. A pause there. The way hope and realism refused to occupy the same hand, no matter how much you tried to hold them both.

A few days before the procedure, Reza called the interventional radiologist to discuss the biopsy. It should have been routine, like any other call about a patient. Instead, it felt like pleading dressed in clinical language.

"Least invasive," the radiologist said. "But highest yield."

They reviewed the images together. One retroperitoneal node met both criteria. When the call ended, Reza sat with the images open on his screen for a moment longer, swallowing back a lump in his throat.

His mother was traveling, and his father had asked that she not be told until she returned. Reza carried that too: the knowing, the waiting, the loneliness of a half-secret kept out of love.

The morning of the biopsy, his phone lit up. His father.

"Maybe we should cancel."

Reza's chest tightened. Not at the words—he understood them—but at what they carried underneath. That fear wasn't irrational. It was honest. His father had spent his life not flinching, and here, finally, was something that made him want to stop.

Reza thought about being five, maybe six. He had been in a kitchen somewhere in Austin, watching his father work at a Burger King while the smell of grease rose through the air. Long days, longer nights, all while earning his PhD in civil engineering after immigrating from Iran. From him, Reza learned what hard work looked like. Steady. Unspoken.

A muffled sound on the line broke Reza out of his swirling thoughts. "Why?" he asked, once his rational mind turned back on.

"What if they hit something important?" his father's voice rang through. "What if it shows something we don't want to know?"

He was not afraid of the needle. He was afraid of the answer. Of the moment after, when the world had to reorganize itself around whatever the results revealed.

"Dad," Reza said, "you're still a very young seventy-two-year-old man." He meant it. He needed him to hear it. "Knowing what's going on, that's the first step. That's how we make sure everything happens the way you want it to."

He told his father that he'd spoken with the interventional radiologist. That the specialist felt confident about the procedure. That the node they'd chosen was accessible, low risk, and that they had been careful selecting it.

There was a pause on the line. Long enough that Reza waited, rather than filling it.

In the end, his father went through with the procedure.

The hours that followed moved strangely. Reza tried to occupy himself the way people did when waiting on something they couldn't accelerate. He played a round of golf, spent an hour on a video game, and even tried to read a few articles. None of it held for long.

In some quiet way, not knowing felt safer. As long as the phone stayed silent, the story hadn't turned.

Then, as his eyes began to blur over another article, his phone buzzed. It was the interventional radiologist.

"Preliminary impression looks lymphoid."

Reza's heart pounded.

Lymphoid. Not carcinoma.

If it had been carcinoma spread this widely, the prognosis would have been grim. But lymphoma opened a different door entirely. He and Rabih had talked it through before the biopsy, turning over the possibilities in a comforting way that made no difference. An indolent lymphoma could look exactly like this—nodes everywhere, yet the patient might feel almost entirely normal.

Relief came, sudden and disorienting. It wasn't good news exactly, but it was the best version of the bad news he'd imagined himself receiving.

Once he steadied himself, he texted Rabih.

Pause and Reflect

With diffuse retroperitoneal and inguinal lymphadenopathy, normal labs, minimal symptoms, and a lymphoid preliminary read, what is most likely?

The pattern fit lymphoma. But the pattern was only half of it, tempo being the other half. Aggressive or indolent.

Five days had passed since the radiologist's call, and each one felt longer than the last.

Reza, once again, tried to stay busy. Work filled the hours in the way it always did. Patients, notes, emails. He even dragged himself out to play a few holes of golf with friends. Still, the uncertainty followed him everywhere, brushing the edges of each moment like a shadow he couldn't shake.

Reza was standing on a fairway, club in hand, when his father texted.

"Results are up."

Time seemed to stretch in slow waves as he stared at the screen. The sun was hitting his forearms like a brand, and he could just barely register the thwacking sound of golf balls behind him. Shaking himself from his stupor, he stepped off the grass toward the cart path and logged into the portal.

He had opened thousands of results over the course of his career. Board scores. Match results. Patient labs. Pathology reports that appeared on a screen and rearranged someone's life in an instant.

None had ever felt like this.

The report loaded slowly. And then the words were there, unmistakable, plain as anything: *consistent with indolent lymphoma.*

Reza read the sentence again. Then again. The sun was still on his forearms; the golf course was still moving around him. The world had continued, indifferent and unchanged, while something inside him went very quiet.

There was only one thing to do.

He FaceTimed his father. The call was answered almost immediately, and his parents' faces filled the screen, calm and curious, waiting. Reza opened his mouth. His throat tightened in a way he hadn't anticipated, tears coming before words could.

"همه چیز اوکی است" he managed. *Everything is okay.*

Then he explained the results to his parents, describing them in detail.

Indolent lymphoma was not benign. But it was manageable, often slow. Sometimes observed without treatment for years. It was the best version of a bad diagnosis.

They listened without interrupting. His father nodded slowly, eyes filling with tears. His mother began to cry. She leaned in and kissed her husband on the cheek.

Later, his father met with a lymphoma expert who confirmed what Reza and Rabih had suspected. The disease appeared indolent, and the specialist explained that treatment was not urgent. Rituximab could reduce the already low lifetime risk of transformation into an aggressive lymphoma, but there was certainly time to think.

Then the doctor asked about his life. About what mattered to him.

My father told him about Los Angeles. A month-long trip he'd been planning to take after retirement. Something he had been looking forward to for years but had begun to worry he might never take. He talked about the places he wanted to see, about the time he wanted to spend with family.

The doctor smiled. "Go to Los Angeles," he said. "Enjoy your trip. When you come back, we can decide whether to treat or observe. There's no rush."

That night, Reza's father called him again.

His voice was different. Lighter. There was something in it that Reza hadn't heard in weeks: excitement, almost disbelief. He spoke about the visit, the reassurance, the plan.

"I think I'm still going to LA," he said.

Something moved through Reza. A wide, warm wave of relief. Not just relief at the pathology, though that was present too, but at the sense that life hadn't reorganized itself. It could continue moving forward.

He sat quietly with the strangeness of what the last couple of weeks had been. At some point along the way, without either of them naming it, the roles had reversed. The man who spent four decades at the same engineering firm, commuting two hours each day just so Reza could attend a strong public high school, had needed reassurance from his son.

And somehow, Reza had been able to offer it. Not as a physician, exactly. But as a son who happened to know enough to help, which was a different and heavier thing entirely.

Only after they hung up did he text Rabih. He called within seconds.

Reza relayed the results, and they fell into a brief silence as the news settled between them. In that silence, Reza felt how dread and gratitude could sit side by side. Intertwined, uncomfortably close.

"Okay," Rabih said finally. Quietly. In a way that meant everything. "We can work with this."

Recap

- When approaching diffuse lymphadenopathy, first ask whether the answer can be reached with blood tests; if not, pursue the safest node that also offers the highest pathologic yield. It must meet both criteria.

- In lymphadenopathy, location and distribution are decisive filters. Retroperitoneal nodes should elevate concern for malignancy even in the absence of symptoms or abnormal labs.

- Physicians should not try to be doctors for their own families. But they cannot remain silent either. Finding that narrow line between guidance and overreach is one of the hardest balances in medicine.

18

They were at a hospital holiday party, plates balanced on paper napkins, cinnamon in the air. *"Last Christmas"* blared from the speakers while they argued about the greatest Christmas song of all time.

Rabih was wearing a sweater with Naar stitched beside a crooked tree. Reza's shirt had Sid and Geno dressed as Santa. They were both carrying the rapid response and code pager, the weight of it familiar against their hips.

The saccharine music continued to swell, blurring the edges of everything: softening the fluorescent lights, the clatter of cutlery, the low hum of conversation. For a moment, the world felt awash in warmth—untouchable. Then the intercom cut in.

"Rapid response. 4E. Room 22."

At the same time, their pagers erupted, slicing through the chorus. They met each other's gaze. No words. They were already moving toward the hallway.

A man in his late fifties sat upright in bed, lips swollen, saliva pooling, eyes fixed on something beyond the room. A wash of dusky blue spread across his mouth—the kind of color that warned before alarms did.

The monitor screamed.

70%.

60%.

56%.

His pulse was present. His blood pressure unremarkable. But his oxygen saturation continued to drop.

Reza moved to the bedside and gripped the man's shoulders. "Sir, can you hear me? Can you speak?" He shook him once, firmly. Not a flinch, not a blink. Just those vacant, unseeing eyes.

He took a quick inventory: airway closing, oxygen low. Non-rebreather. Suction. Respiratory therapy.

The patient's oxygen saturation climbed—fifty-seven, fifty-eight—then stopped.

The possibility of losing the pulse sharpened. Reza ran through the steps: bed down, backboard ready, fingers already moving toward the carotid.

Rabih's hand hovered over the code button. His mind ran through the teaching cemented from experience and lectures alike: it was better to be loud and wrong than silent and too late. And when in doubt, ask someone in the room.

It took one sharp nod from Reza to finalize his decision. The response came like a wave: ICU, pharmacy, respiratory therapy, residents, nurses. A surge of bodies and urgency, followed by the inevitable extras drawn by instinct more than purpose.

Within thirty seconds of the code being called, the patient's pulse disappeared. Those without a role drifted toward the bed, pulled by gravity and adrenaline, unsure whether to step in or step back.

Rabih's eyes scanned the room. Too many bodies. Too much sound. Communication fraying at the edges. "I'm leading," he spoke up, voice steady and cutting through the noise. "I need everyone to be quiet. If you don't have a purpose, step out."

Roles were briskly assigned: compressions, airway, access, medications, and time.

Pads went on.

"Rhythm?"

"PEA."

In the corner of Reza's vision, an IV pole hung with ferric carboxymaltose.

"He started itching right after the infusion," the nurse said, following Reza's gaze.

Swollen lips, hypoxia, infusion. The pieces locked together.

"We need one milligram of epi, IV push," Reza called out as he moved to sub in for the person performing compressions.

The nurse checked the line. "The IV isn't flowing."

In arrest, unreliable access was no access.

"Then we need IOs," Rabih ordered.

Two IOs went in. Compressions never stopped, the steady thrum of hands and bodies echoing through the room. Time seemed to stretch, elastic and heavy, each two-minute cycle long enough to hold its own fear.

Between compressions, Rabih studied the man's face. Late fifties. Too young. Swollen lips, eyes empty, a life caught between moments. He thought of all the families he had been forced to wake with bad news. If it went that way, this would be one of the harder ones.

A pulse flickered beneath his fingers, weak and uncertain. It vanished. Then returned. A fragile victory. The tube slid in smoothly, pressors were started, and a rhythm finally stabilized on the monitor. For a moment, the room held—quiet, stunned, alive.

Then the intercom cut in once more.

"Rapid response. 9S. Bed 21."

At the same moment, their pagers erupted again. The same insistence, a different emergency.

Rabih didn't look away from the bed, still tracking every rise and fall of the patient's chest. "Break off. Go."

Reza peeled toward the door.

The next room was calmer in a way that didn't quite feel like peace. A ninety-four-year-old woman with advanced dementia lay in bed, her body a record of every intervention that had been made on her behalf. A tracheostomy collar, a G-tube, a suprapubic catheter. She was unresponsive, not with the electric absence of the man a few floors down, but as if the night had simply settled too heavily on her.

Her blood pressure and oxygen saturation were normal.

Her temperature was 92°F.

Pause and Reflect

What is your approach to hypothermia?

Hypothermia reflects either excessive heat loss or impaired heat production, and the clinical context usually clarifies which mechanism is most likely.

Figure 18.1

Differential Diagnosis of Hypothermia

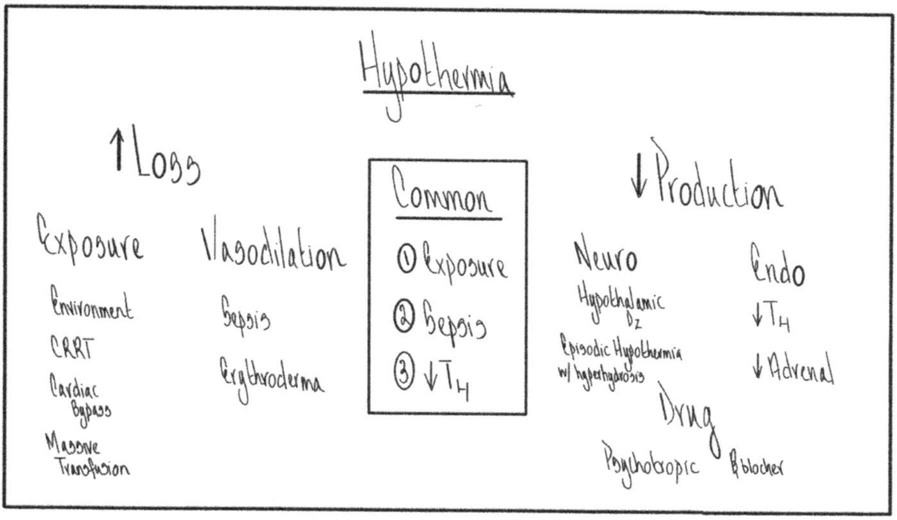

Hypothermia most commonly results from excessive heat loss or impaired heat production, with infection representing a frequent cause in hospitalized patients.

Reza glanced around the bed, locking eyes with the nurse, the residents, and the respiratory therapist.

A resident stepped forward and delivered the one-liner. "Ninety-four-year-old woman, full code, in and out of the ICU. Follows commands at baseline."

"She's ninety-four and hospitalized," Reza said, approaching the patient. "Hypothermia is infection until proven otherwise."

He gestured toward the monitor without urgency, as if inviting the team to think alongside him. "Older patients don't mount fevers. A small pneumonia, early sepsis, or even a slight physiologic hit could show up as confusion and cold skin instead of heat."

"We need a fingerstick glucose, EKG, blood cultures, CBC, and lactate. Empiric vanc-zosyn."

One resident added, "Cortisol and TSH. And a CT head."

Another glanced up. "She's been here a while. Should we start with meropenem because of ESBL risk factors?"

Reza nodded. "Let's do it."

Over the next few days, the patient stabilized enough to move to step-down.

Reza sat at the computer as her results began to populate the screen one by one.

Normal CT head. Normal TSH and cortisol. White count unimpressive.

The story should have been infection. The pieces pointed that way, and he had followed them without pause. But something in the results resisted the script, a quiet incongruence that couldn't yet be named.

Pause and Reflect

What blood test are you eagerly awaiting?

The blood gas appeared.

pH 7.1. PCO_2 120. Every frozen inch of skin whispered what the labs confirmed: she was drowning from the inside, slowly and silently.

The picture, once studied, had its own logic. A mild infection in a woman this fragile didn't need dramatics. It only had to trigger encephalopathy, leading to hypoventilation and severe hypercapnia. Then the cycle tightened: the cold that had triggered alarm was not the cause but the consequence—a reinforcing loop of hypercapnia, hypothermia, worsened mental status, and worsened ventilation.

Severe hypercapnia reflects inadequate ventilation.

Figure 18.2

Causes of Hypoventilation

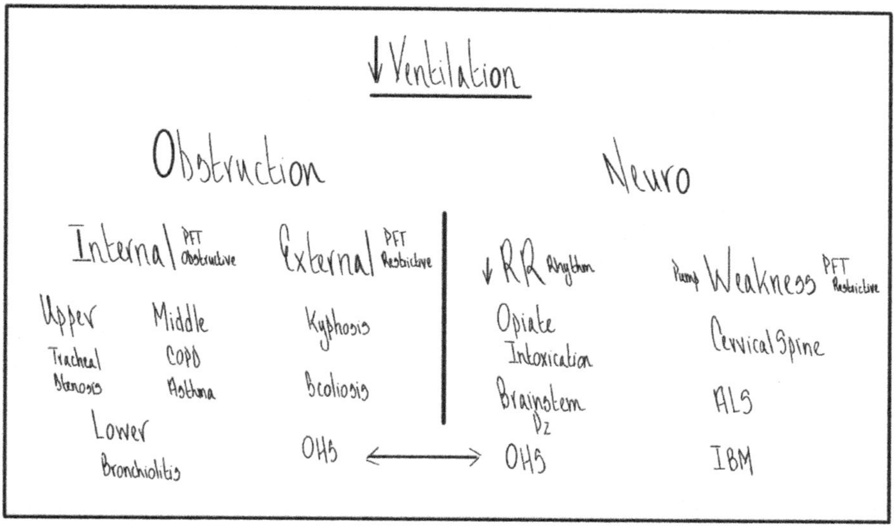

Hypoventilation results from airway obstruction, impaired chest wall mechanics, depressed central respiratory drive, or neuromuscular weakness, each leading to carbon dioxide retention.

The ventilator connected to the trach with a soft click. Reza stood back and watched. It took mere minutes for the woman's eyelids to flutter. Her eyes opened.

Pseudomonas later appeared in the sputum culture, but that night, hypercapnia was the true enemy.

The first patient was extubated the day after his cardiac arrest. He tried to pull the tube out even earlier, irritated by the plastic insisting on its place.

The second patient woke as soon as the carbon dioxide cleared, the infection real but secondary to the slow suffocation that had stolen her consciousness.

Days later, Rabih and Reza sat at Rabih's kitchen counter, bowls of açai between them. Rabih sprinkled granola with the seriousness of a proceduralist adjusting a line. Reza watched with a look of mock reverence, as if he, too, understood the physics of texture.

"That's too much," Reza said finally.

Rabih didn't look up. "No such thing."

The conversation settled from there, easy and familiar. It drifted in slow loops between work and family life and work again. They did not talk about heroics. They talked about the moments the rooms fell quiet. About the blood gas that shifted the night.

Medicine was rarely about the dramatic saves. Most nights, it was repetition. Compressions that blurred together, a lab value that changed everything, an airway secured before hesitation had time to grow.

That was the true work. Not the heroics. The repetition. The willingness to return.

Recap

- Anaphylaxis from IV iron is real but rare; a single adverse event should not distort appropriate prescribing when the base rate supports benefit.

- In hospitalized patients, hypothermia is infection until proven otherwise, but ventilation must always be assessed. Severe hypercapnia can lower temperature and alter mental status more dramatically than the infection itself.

- Running a code requires a leader who quiets the room, invites focused input, and assigns clear roles, creating the psychological safety that allows a team to perform under pressure.

19

Rabih started his morning the way he usually did. Coffee first.

He moved quietly because Reza was asleep in his guest room. It was his birthday—forty, which felt like something worth acknowledging.

Rabih ground the coffee beans softer than usual and closed the cabinets with both hands. At one point he thought about letting Naar, his dog, do what Naar usually did, which was make enough noise to wake anyone within three units of the apartment building. Just so Naar could be the first to say happy birthday. Instead, he let Reza sleep.

But Naar, upon hearing the neighbor's tiny dog, his sworn nemesis, had other plans. He released one sharp, decisive bark. Rabih, sitting on the sofa with coffee and a book in hand, did not rush to stop him. He continued to read quietly, no phone in sight. Just pages and the early light streaming through the windows.

He heard socks against hardwood about twenty minutes later. Reza came down the hallway, hair undecided, eyes half open.

Rabih stood and opened his arms. "Forty. Wow."

Reza walked into it. "Be gentle."

They laced up and headed toward Runyon Canyon before the morning could shift into day. The early hour brought cool air and silence, a welcome sort of slowness.

"It's just a light jog, right?" Reza asked. It landed as more of a plea than a question.

"Flat. Scenic. Gentle."

The first corner tilted upward into a steep hill. The kind that functioned as a cheap cardiac stress test.

Reza didn't say anything for a moment, but when he spoke, he was out of breath. "You planned this."

Rabih lengthened his stride, flashing a grin in Reza's direction. "I have no idea what you're talking about."

After the run, Rabih made açai. He bought it in bulk and measured it to the gram, because who would he be if not meticulous? Reza raised an eyebrow at the kitchen scale but said nothing. He finished the bowl without complaint.

Soon after, they sank into the apartment building jacuzzi that resided on the rooftop, giving them a clear view of the LA skyline. The jets flared to life, then settled. Rabih handed over a lime LaCroix.

"You've been quiet," Reza said, scanning his face with suspicious eyes.

Rabih looked at him, lips lifting at the corners. "I have a case for you."

"It better be good. It's my birthday."

"It starts in an OR. A sixty-seven-year-old woman getting an elective rhinoplasty. She's sedated and intubated. Then she loses her pulse."

"PEA?"

"PEA. Two rounds of CPR. Two milligrams of epinephrine. ROSC. Now she's in our ED."

Pause and Reflect

She regained a pulse after PEA arrest. What is your differential?

When cardiac arrest occurs with electrical activity but no pulse, the diagnostic task is to rapidly separate microscopic causes from macroscopic ones.

Figure 19.1
PEA Arrest

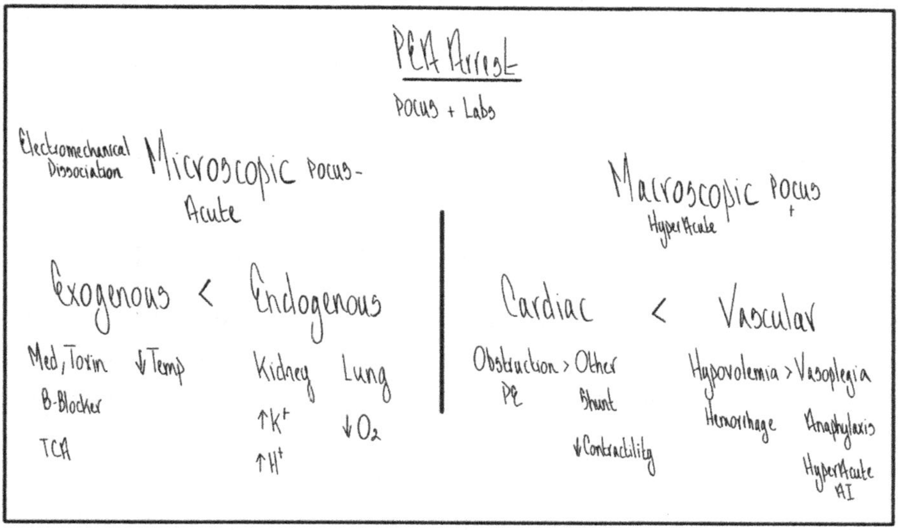

Pulseless electrical activity reflects either microscopic causes of electromechanical dissociation or macroscopic circulatory collapse detectable with a focused ultrasound and laboratory data.

When Rabih thought about PEA, he still respected the Hs and Ts. But over time, he started using a tighter frame.

PEA was shock so severe that the pulse disappeared. That reframe made the question simpler: what shock state could erase the pulse?

Obstructive causes rose first. Tamponade. Tension pneumothorax. Massive pulmonary embolism.

Then distributive states. Anaphylaxis, especially in the peri-intubation window.

Hypovolemia belonged there too. Sudden hemorrhage or rapid volume loss.

Then the lens widened further. Metabolic collapse and toxins, hyperkalemia, severe acidosis, medication effects. These were not classic shock states, but they could extinguish perfusion just as completely.

Reza had been listening with his arms resting on the lip of the jacuzzi. "So you were translating rhythm into physiology."

"Exactly. PEA isn't a rhythm puzzle. It's a perfusion puzzle."

It was a useful frame, but it was also one that revealed the blind spots in Rabih's reasoning. Three assumptions had quietly crept in.

The first was assuming PEA meant noncardiac. Cardiogenic processes absolutely landed in PEA, especially when the mechanism was bradycardia or conduction block rather than ventricular tachyarrhythmia.

The second was reflexively equating ST elevation with plaque rupture and stopping there. That reflex was strong and typically sound, but pulmonary embolism, myopericarditis, and Takotsubo could all produce similar patterns on an EKG.

The third assumption was harder to name. It would only reveal itself later, once the story had fully unfolded.

The patient's post-ROSC EKG had shown inferior ST elevations with reciprocal changes and complete heart block. She was stabilized at the bedside while the cath lab mobilized. But her coronary angiogram was pristine. There was no evidence of coronary obstruction.

Reza dunked his head beneath the water, staying there for a beat before resurfacing.

“That’s not allowed.”

“I know,” Rabih said. “But it happened.”

Pause and Reflect

How can the cath be negative if she truly had ischemia?

Not every acute coronary syndrome reveals a culprit lesion on angiography.

Figure 19.2
Cath-Negative ACS

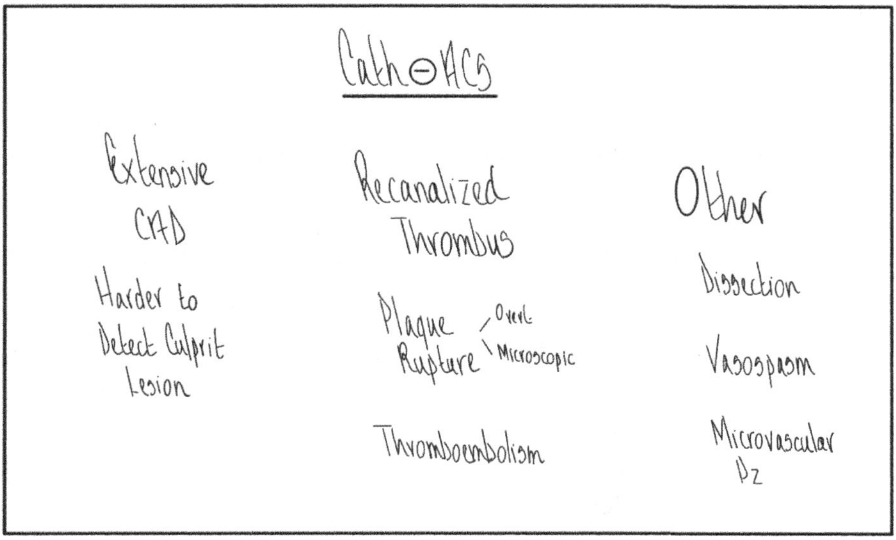

When angiography does not show an obstructive coronary lesion, the differential diagnosis includes plaque disruption with recanalization, coronary spasm, dissection, and microvascular disease.

The third assumption that made his reasoning vulnerable was that a normal angiogram ended the story. It didn't.

A clean picture could still hide dynamic vascular behavior. Recanalized thrombus. Coronary vasospasm. Microvascular dysfunction. Coronary dissection.

Ten hours later, the patient's EKG was normal. Then her chest pain returned. And with it came the same ST elevations—the same pattern, the same fear.

Nitroglycerin was given, and the pain resolved. The EKG normalized again.

Reza locked the frame into place. "Inter-episodic."

"Exactly. Abnormal, normal. Abnormal. Nitro responsive."

Pause and Reflect

What is the final diagnosis?

"So what was it?" Reza asked, shielding his eyes from the sun.

Rabih watched him. "Mechanism. Dynamic vascular behavior, not fixed plaque."

Coronary vasospasm. Reversible constriction that behaved like an occlusion and disappeared before the camera arrived.

The echo showed apical ballooning with basal hyperkinesis. Features consistent with stress cardiomyopathy. Vasospasm and Takotsubo shared the same catecholamine engine, which put them in overlap territory. Peri-intubation autonomic swings, epinephrine during resuscitation, hyperventilation. All feeding the same surge.

Which left three questions: what triggered it, how to prevent recurrence, and what to do differently when the patient faced anesthesia again.

They treated with calcium channel blockers and nitrates. Then they went through her history for triggers: tobacco, stimulants, vasoconstrictive medications. They counseled her carefully about future procedures and autonomic volatility.

She walked out of the hospital after five days.

The bubbles in the jacuzzi had gone quiet while they were talking. The jets had timed out, and the surface became something flat and still.

Rabih reached over and pressed the button again. The water roared back to life.

"You know what I like about this case?" he asked.

Reza waited.

"You can't read it from a single frame. You have to watch the movement, the transitions. The space between touches."

Recap

- PEA is not a rhythm problem; it is a perfusion problem. Translate the arrest into physiology before chasing labels.
- Tempo matters. An inter-episodic pattern of ST elevation that normalizes with nitroglycerin should narrow the frame toward vasospasm.

20

The night started in one language and ended in another.

A French family clustered around a stretcher, speaking quickly, translating in fragments. Between them sat an elderly woman who looked smaller than her resume suggested. The family said she was an executive, still working, still sharp, until three days ago. Now she was nauseated, vomiting, and slightly disoriented.

Someone held out a scrap of paper with home blood pressure readings on it, offered like evidence. A single number was highlighted in yellow: *systolic 192.*

It was the kind of presentation that made the mind search for a single unifying emergency: nausea, vomiting, confusion, hypertension. Something in the head? Intracranial catastrophe. Hemorrhage. Mass effect. A lesion that made the combination of vomiting and confusion teach us fear. The consequence of missing it could be irreversible.

When hypertension presents with acute neurologic symptoms, first distinguish vascular emergencies from parenchymal causes of increased intracranial pressure.

Figure 20.1

Acute Hypertension with Neurologic Symptoms

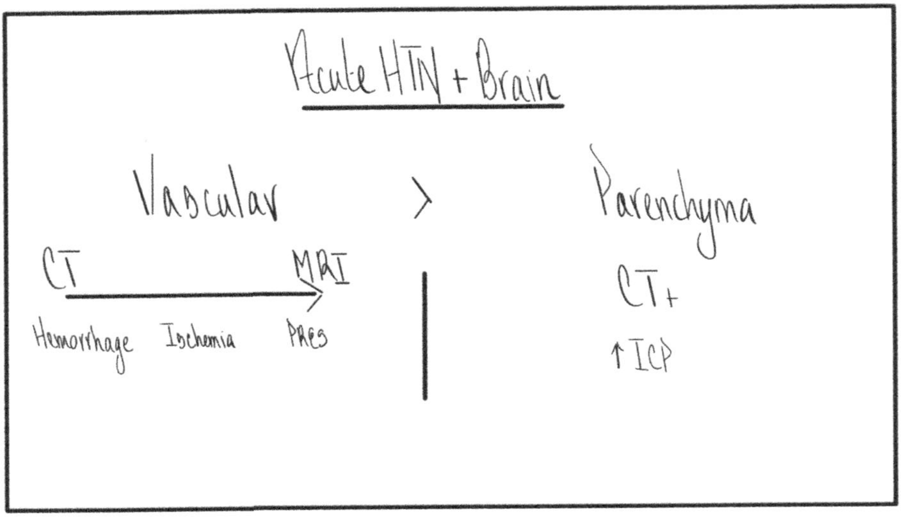

Acute hypertension with neurologic symptoms should first prompt evaluation for intracranial vascular emergencies before considering parenchymal processes that increase intracranial pressure.

The history was difficult to obtain.

It was the middle of the night, so there was no on-site interpreter. The patient was confused. The family was doing their best, but nuance blurred when language was strained and everyone was afraid. Voices spoke over each other, one sentence interrupting another. A correction followed every question. Someone gestured toward the patient, then toward the hallway, then back at Reza and Rabih. Worry made everything urgent at once.

So they did what they could do well. They stabilized, examined, and let the early data steer toward the safest branch.

From the family, they pieced together that the patient's nausea preceded the blood pressure spike. She had been unable to keep anything down, which meant she stopped taking her antihypertensives. Then the home cuff caught the number, and the number became the headline.

That detail mattered. Not because hypertension was benign, but because sometimes it was downstream of the story rather than its cause.

The CT head came back quickly. Unrevealing. Then a lab returned that made them pause.

Sodium: 110.

Reza looked at Rabih in their workroom, twirling a pen between his fingers. "That's the culprit."

A sodium of 110 did not politely enter the differential. It took over the bay. Now the nausea, vomiting, confusion—even the hypertension—shifted in tone.

Hyponatremia reflects an excess of water relative to sodium, most commonly mediated through antidiuretic hormone activity.

Figure 20.2

Mechanisms of Hyponatremia

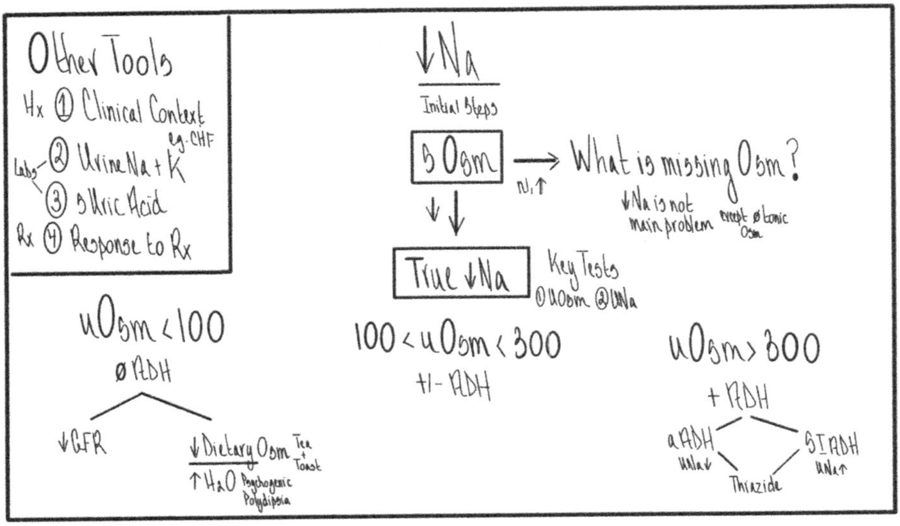

Hyponatremia most often results from antidiuretic hormone–mediated water retention, and urine osmolality and urine sodium help determine whether ADH activity is absent, appropriate, or inappropriate.

As more labs came through, the blood pressure began to look less like a culprit and more like a bystander.

Creatinine 0.76, anion gap 17, glucose normal. Urinalysis with a specific gravity of 1.017. Two-plus ketones. Serum alcohol undetectable. The numbers arrived in pieces, and each one quietly narrowed the frame.

Hyponatremia often looked manageable—the numbers responded, and the branches seemed clear. But that clarity could be deceiving. So they slowed down and asked the questions that took precedence.

First: was this hypotonic? By base rate, almost certainly. Still, they checked a serum osmolality because pseudohyponatremia and hypertonic states were predictable traps, too easy to overlook.

Second: was ADH active? The urine wasn't dilute, and a specific gravity of 1.017 meant the kidneys were holding on to water—evidence that ADH was on.

Third: was the ADH response appropriate or inappropriate? The next labs answered. A high urine sodium of 65 and a very low serum uric acid of 1.8 showed the kidneys behaving as if volume were adequate, pointing towards persistent ADH activity when it should have been off.

Concentrated urine, high urine sodium, low serum uric acid. Taken separately, each was a data point. Together, they told a coherent story.

Pause and Reflect

How would you label the hyponatremia?

SIADH.

Urine sodium could be used as a proxy for aldosterone activity. If aldosterone was active, urine sodium tended to be low. If it was high—without diuretics, renal failure, or fluid confounders—it was labeled as SIADH physiology.

But what caused the lower serum uric acid?

In SIADH, excess ADH led to free-water retention and subtle expansion of effective intravascular volume. That expansion increased urinary uric acid loss and suppressed aldosterone, allowing serum uric acid to remain low and urine sodium to remain high.

The patient received intravenous fluids, a reflex that felt kind and safe in a vomiting patient. Within hours, her sodium climbed from 110 to 124.

Reza exhaled, studying the number. "That's too fast."

When sodium rose that quickly, the priority shifted. There was a need to prevent osmotic demyelination and to reverse overcorrection. The precise risk from any single correction rate was debated, and ODS was rare, but in severe hyponatremia, rapid osmotic shifts were injuries that were still preventable.

Pause and Reflect

How would you label the hyponatremia after it increased with fluid?

True SIADH typically worsened with isotonic fluid because free water was retained while sodium was excreted in concentrated urine.

But this patient improved. Dramatically. That behavior fit hypovolemia. When volume was restored, ADH turned off, free water was excreted, and the sodium rose.

Now they sat with that tension.

The urine studies whispered SIADH. The clinical response shouted volume depletion.

Real cases refused to be clean. Mechanisms overlapped, and some etiologies, especially thiazides, impersonated both worlds.

So they pulled the thread that mattered most: medications.

Not just what she was taking, but what lurked inside the combination pill. What had been unchanged for years. What was missed when the history passed through fear and language barriers.

She was on lisinopril–hydrochlorothiazide. The lisinopril surfaced early. The thiazide arrived later, only after someone recalled the exact tablet.

Now the physiology aligned. Thiazide-associated hyponatremia could mimic SIADH—high urine sodium, low serum uric acid—even though thiazides typically raised uric acid. ADH-driven physiology had masked the underlying volume depletion but corrected briskly once volume was restored and the drug was stopped.

With the picture clear, they moved decisively. They gave DDAVP and D5W, carefully re-lowering the sodium, with nephrology at the bedside rather than just on the chart.

They watched her closely. Time passed, measured and quiet. No delayed neurologic collapse, no osmotic demyelination. She improved, and when she left the hospital days later, it was with a new understanding—of the medication, of the physiology, and of what had nearly been missed.

As Rabih and Reza stepped out of the room, the family thanked them in French—voices steadier now, fear replaced by something quieter.

Merci, docteur.

They answered simply.

De rien.

Recap

- When nausea, vomiting, confusion, and hypertension coexist, first exclude intracranial catastrophe before assigning causality to the blood pressure.
- The response of plasma sodium to fluids is often more informative than a single urine study when ADH physiology is uncertain.
- Limited shared language should slow interpretation, not accelerate conclusions.

21

The room was dark despite it being morning. The shades were drawn, and the covers were pulled over the patient's head, as if she had decided overnight that the world could wait. Reza and Rabih knocked softly and asked if they could come in.

She lowered the blanket just enough to show her face. It was weary, withdrawn—older than the number in the chart by an immeasurable amount of years. The kind of tired that sleep didn't touch.

She was far from home. Her children had flown her here because they could see what she could not, or perhaps what she refused to: she was fading. Quietly, steadily, the way a candle died out when no one was watching.

"Doc, I'm just… exhausted. I'm weak. And I keep falling."

They listened. Then they looked.

At first glance, her abdomen looked distended in a way that didn't belong to the rest of her body. It sat atop a shrinking frame.

Her outside records hadn't arrived yet. So with no history to lean on and no prior chart to consult, they started from scratch.

The patient offered three symptoms: fatigue, weakness, and frequent falls.

Pause and Reflect

Which symptom gives the most diagnostic leverage?

Fatigue, by itself, rarely did. It signaled that something was wrong, sometimes profoundly so, but not where or what. Weakness was more promising, but it was a word that had to be earned. Before it helped, it must be clarified.

But falls were different. Falls were events. They happened in time and space, and they left something to interrogate.

So Rabih and Reza began there.

When clinicians heard the word "fall," they often reflexively asked about loss of consciousness. Transient loss of consciousness opened specific doors: syncope, seizure, hypoglycemia, and, rarely, strategic strokes.

But most falls didn't fit into that category. Most were labeled "mechanical," a term too often treated as a terminal diagnosis. A way of saying *nothing to see here.* That was a mistake. "Mechanical" was a proximal description, not an explanation. It described how someone fell, not why they were vulnerable in the first place. When that question went unasked, both the diagnosis and the opportunity to prevent the next fall were missed.

The patient explained that when she stood, she felt unable to hold herself upright. She didn't lose consciousness or feel dizzy. She described it more like imbalance and collapse.

Her orthostatic vitals were checked. They were positive, confirmed by her symptoms and by a drop in systolic pressure.

Then came the detail that shifted the frame: her blood pressure fell as expected, but her heart rate did not rise to compensate. It held steady—a clue.

The pattern of heart rate response during orthostatic hypotension often reveals the underlying mechanism.

Figure 21.1

Orthostasis Clues

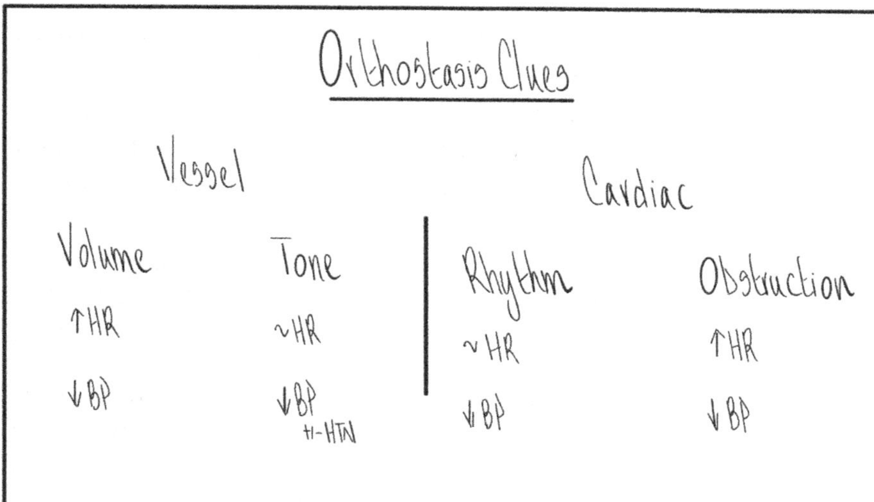

The heart rate response during orthostatic hypotension helps distinguish volume depletion from autonomic failure or cardiac causes.

Rabih looked at the monitor, then at Reza. The patient was watching both of them, tracking their expressions with her eyes.

"Not volume," Rabih said quietly.

Reza nodded. "No. Not volume."

What had seemed straightforward began to take on a different shape. Without compensatory tachycardia, the differential moved toward autonomic insufficiency, including medications, neurodegenerative disease, and infiltrative processes like amyloidosis.

They held that thought but turned back to the patient, asking about her weakness.

She described exhaustion even at rest. Lying in bed, she felt depleted, and movement only made it worse.

That distinction mattered. True neurologic motor weakness declared itself when muscles were asked to work. What she described was different: a global reduction in energy and stamina that worsened with exertion, rather than revealing a focal loss of strength. This pattern pointed away from primary neuromuscular disease and toward systems that failed under demand: cardiopulmonary, vascular, or global metabolic processes. The term *asthenia* was sometimes used to describe this pervasive lack of energy rather than focal weakness. And while the word was uncommon outside of medical texts, the experience was not.

At this stage, her fatigue remained nonspecific. What gave it meaning was when it appeared and what made it worse. That temporal relationship quietly aligned with a cardiopulmonary or systemic limitation—something that would later help organize the rest of the patient's story.

Their clinical reasoning had begun to drift from the bedside, but Rabih's attention returned to the patient. Her abdomen kept drawing his focus. It was enough to pursue an ultrasound, revealing free fluid. Ascites.

The discovery shifted the frame once again. With new-onset ascites, two questions mattered more than anything else.

Pause and Reflect

What are those two questions?

1. What was the SAAG?
2. Was the ascitic fluid infected?

Everything else could wait.

The patient mentioned, almost in passing, that a CT scan at her hometown hospital was read as *"cirrhotic-appearing liver."* But radiographic cirrhosis was exactly that: a radiographic impression. Imaging alone did not establish cirrhosis, and it was commonly overcalled, especially in the presence of ascites.

Before the outside scan arrived, her labs returned. Platelets around 500,000, hemoglobin 8.8, white count mildly elevated. Her INR, bilirubin, and AST and ALT were normal.

A platelet count that high practically excluded cirrhosis as the explanation for her ascites. Portal hypertension did not coexist comfortably with thrombocytosis.

Rabih scanned the labs again, eyes glued to the platelet count. "That's not cirrhosis."

Reza exhaled. "No. Something else is doing this."

Paracentesis showed a SAAG of 1.1 and a total protein greater than 2.5.

A high SAAG signaled portal hypertension. A low SAAG pointed toward exudative processes such as malignancy. This value sat at the border. They resisted forcing it into either category.

What stood out more was the total protein. In cirrhosis, portal hypertension filtered protein-poor fluid across the hepatic sinusoids, so ascitic protein was usually low. High-protein ascites suggested a different physiology, one seen with cardiac disease or exudative processes.

The heart was evaluated next. Echo normal, BNP normal. So the cardiac branch weakened.

Then the CT chest, abdomen, and pelvis arrived. Omental thickening and nodularity. Peritoneal enhancement. Moderate ascites.

The puzzle shifted. The peritoneum was inflamed. The SAAG of 1.1, previously floating at the border, clicked into place. Imaging showed disease directly on the peritoneal surface, where it could disrupt the endothelium and allow protein-rich fluid to leak into the abdominal cavity.

In retrospect, the high-protein ascites made sense. The problem was no longer cirrhosis. It was an infiltrative disease along the peritoneum.

Pause and Reflect

What is your differential?

Subacute disease involving the peritoneum most often reflects malignancy, granulomatous infection, or less common inflammatory processes.

Figure 21.2

Subacute Peritoneal Disease

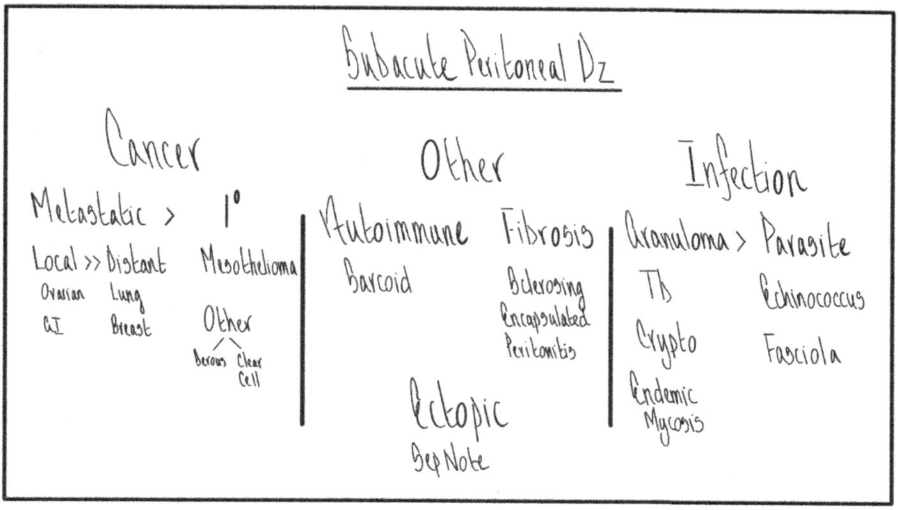

Subacute peritoneal disease is most commonly caused by malignancy, granulomatous infection, or inflammatory disorders affecting the peritoneal surface.

The differential narrowed: infection, autoimmunity, malignancy. Malignancy carried the greatest weight.

By the time outside records arrived, the patient had already undergone an open laparotomy. Surgeons described diffuse nodularity throughout the peritoneum. Biopsies were taken. TB testing was negative.

Ascitic cytology was also negative, a finding that mattered here. While not definitive, it offered reassurance, lowering the probability of metastatic cancer even in the setting of extensive peritoneal disease.

Then another detail surfaced. Forty years ago, during home renovations, she had been exposed to asbestos. Significantly, repeatedly. Long enough to matter.

Some diseases whispered early and shouted later. They lingered, patient in their longevity. Asbestos-related disease belonged to that category—decades of silence, then this.

Pathology reviewed the slides. Primary peritoneal mesothelioma.

In the end, nothing explained why her orthostatics behaved the way they did. Hypotension without tachycardia suggested a blunted baroreflex, consistent with autonomic dysfunction. Whether preexisting, age-related, systemic, or paraneoplastic, the mechanism remained uncertain.

The patient was propped up in the hospital bed, her head resting against a pillow. Rabih and Reza sat beside her in two chairs pulled close to the bedside. The room had grown quiet after the explanation.

Her expression was serious, almost composed. Not the composure of someone who didn't understand, but one of someone who was feeling everything at once and had chosen to hold it very, very carefully. After a moment, she looked directly at them and asked, almost in passing,

"Am I dying?"

The phrasing caught them off guard. It wasn't the question itself but the way she had asked it. *Almost in passing.* As if she were confirming something she had already begun to accept.

They explained that oncology would review the case, that there were treatments to discuss, possibilities to consider. What those treatments might change and what they might not was still uncertain.

She listened without interrupting.

Then she blinked once, still holding their gaze, and asked again,

"Am I dying?"

This time, they didn't cushion their answer.

There was no cure. Available treatments were unlikely to meaningfully alter the course of the disease. How much time she had could not be predicted beyond it no longer being the open question it once was.

Then she asked, "Can you kill me?"

The words didn't land; they sank. Tears formed before thoughts could, and they found themselves kneeling at her bedside, not because they chose to, but because sitting back felt wrong. For a long moment, neither of them spoke. The silence held things that words would only diminish.

The patient was the one who broke it, and she did so gently, with a single tear tracking down her cheek. "I'm not afraid of dying. I just don't want it to be slow." A pause. She swallowed, then went on. "I don't want to be in pain. I would never kill myself. I just want it to be on my terms."

Something settled in the air. Their answer came without defensiveness and without haste. It arose from somewhere much quieter.

No.

They could not end her life. But they could promise her something real, not as a formality and not born of pity. They would stay. They would adjust her medications. Whatever time she had left, pain would not be the loudest thing in the room.

Contact information was exchanged, and care was coordinated. She went home, living out whatever remained in her own space, in her own light, surrounded by what was familiar and loved.

When she died, it was peaceful. Their words had held.

There was no cure for dying. There never would be. But there was presence, and there was relief from suffering, and there was a quiet promise to stay. Sometimes, in medicine, that was the most sacred thing that one person could offer another.

Recap

- When multiple symptoms compete for attention, identify the finding that must be explained. In this case, new-onset ascites organized the rest of the uncertainty.
- Orthostatic hypotension without compensatory tachycardia signals a blunted baroreflex and meaningfully narrows the differential, even when the precise mechanism remains uncertain.
- When a cure is not possible, the work of medicine shifts to presence, symptom control, and dignity; the promise to stay is still a form of treatment.

If this book changed how you think about diagnosis,
a brief review on Amazon helps other clinicians find it.

Stay Connected with *RLRCPSolvers*

If you made it here, thank you.

These cases reflect how we have learned medicine over time—not through certainty, but by revisiting the same questions, challenging our first impressions, and learning to see problems more clearly.

We continue this work each week through *RLRCPSolvers,* where we discuss new cases, build diagnostic frameworks, and share visual tools that help organize clinical problems.

If this approach resonates with you, we would love to continue learning together.

Join the mailing list to receive:

- Summaries of key themes from podcast cases
- Updates on new projects, including our YouTube channel
- Announcements about future books and related work

We don't send emails often, but when we do, it's with intention.

Learn more and sign up at: https://www.rlrcpsolvers.com/newsletter/

Reza and Rabih's Principles of Diagnosis

compiled by Alec and Austin Rezigh

Localization:

- Specify *where* the problem is before investigating *why* it's happening. The more precisely you localize, the more refined your problem representation becomes.

Tempo is queen:

- Diagnosis is like music: the sequence of symptoms and the tempo of disease shape the final interpretation.

Anchor in the base rate:

- Esoteric diagnoses can be exciting—but remember, they're uncommon. Hold rarer causes in reserve so if the expected trajectory fails, you are ready to pivot without delay.

Time is one of the best diagnostic tests:

- Watching the evolution of a clinical syndrome is a powerful tool. But time is fleeting, constantly moving forward. When using time as a test, think of it like an alarm clock: you must schedule it and be ready to reassess when it rings.

The power of problem representation:

- The better you define a problem, the closer you get to solving it. You can't reach the right answer if you're tackling the wrong question. Be patient, ensure understanding, and recognize that the problem representations may evolve over time. As you gather more information or face ongoing uncertainty, update, refine, and reframe your thinking.

Uncertainty is the norm, not the exception:

- Think of uncertainty as a rest stop on your way to a diagnosis, not your final destination. Take a moment—stretch your legs, collect yourself. Then get back in the car. You're still moving forward.

"I don't know" is a strength, not a weakness:

- It's okay not to have an approach at first. Be honest about what you don't know, vocalize it, and grow from it. The only mistake is seeing the same problem twice and not getting better the second time.

The law of proportionality:

- When the depth of an abnormality is out of proportion to the assigned clinical condition, keep searching for more answers.

Reflection, listening, and repetition (RLR):

- RLR doesn't just stand for *Reza loves Rabih*. Reflecting on cases (both the mistakes and the successes), listening intently to your patients and colleagues, and repeating this cycle are the key ingredients to sharpening your diagnostic skills.

APPENDIX

Expanded Figure Legends

These expanded figure legends are designed to highlight the core teaching principles of each topic. They are not intended to provide a comprehensive differential diagnosis or full pathophysiologic review. For deeper exploration, readers are encouraged to engage with additional resources such as RLR (rlrcpsolvers.com) and The Clinical Problem Solvers (clinicalproblemsolving.com).

Figure 1.1
Diagnostic Approach to Pharyngitis

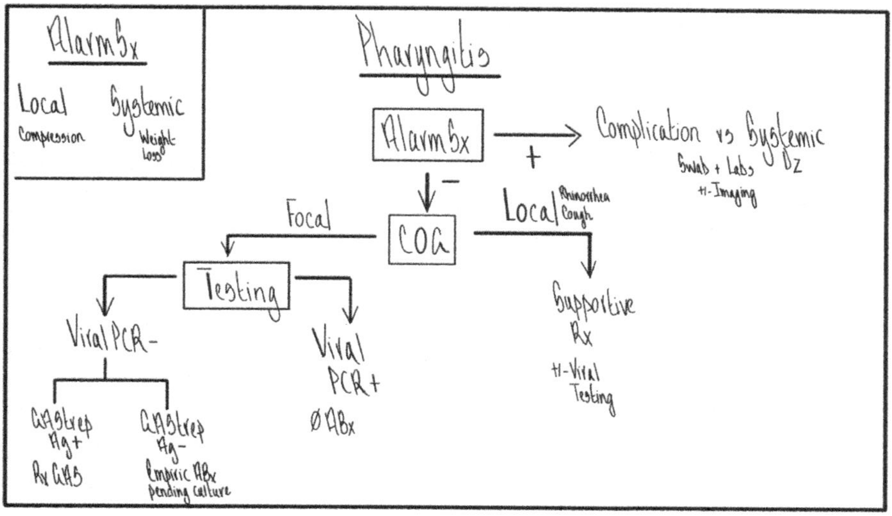

Our approach to pharyngitis begins with a focused search for alarm features—local findings such as dysphagia or dysphonia, and systemic features such as weight loss. The presence of any alarm symptom prompts immediate escalation, including airway assessment and consideration of neck imaging, to evaluate for suppurative complications or other serious pathology.

In the absence of alarm features, the next step is syndromic classification. We distinguish between focal pharyngitis (throat-centered inflammation without prominent cough, rhinorrhea, or myalgias) and diffuse viral syndromes, which involve broader upper respiratory symptoms. Diffuse presentations are managed supportively with targeted viral testing, whereas focal syndromes trigger a structured diagnostic pathway.

For focal pharyngitis, evaluation proceeds stepwise. Viral testing (e.g., influenza, RSV, COVID-19) is performed first, as a positive result typically explains the syndrome and limits further testing. If viral studies are negative, rapid antigen testing for *Group A Streptococcus* (GAS) follows, with antibiotic therapy indicated for positive results. Negative antigen testing is confirmed with throat culture to evaluate for GAS and other bacterial pathogens.

When both viral and GAS testing are negative and suspicion for bacterial infection persists—particularly with prolonged symptoms, atypical features, or high-risk exposures—broader antibacterial coverage may be considered, including treatment targeting anaerobic organisms such as *Fusobacterium*.

Throughout the evaluation, clinicians should remain attentive to sexually transmitted infections, including syphilis, gonorrhea, chlamydia, and HIV, in patients with relevant risk factors. These etiologies often fall outside traditional clinical scoring systems and require targeted history and nucleic acid testing.

This framework prioritizes early identification of dangerous conditions, followed by syndromic classification and stepwise testing, while remaining adaptable to the clinical context.

Figure 1.2
Suppurative Complications of Pharyngitis

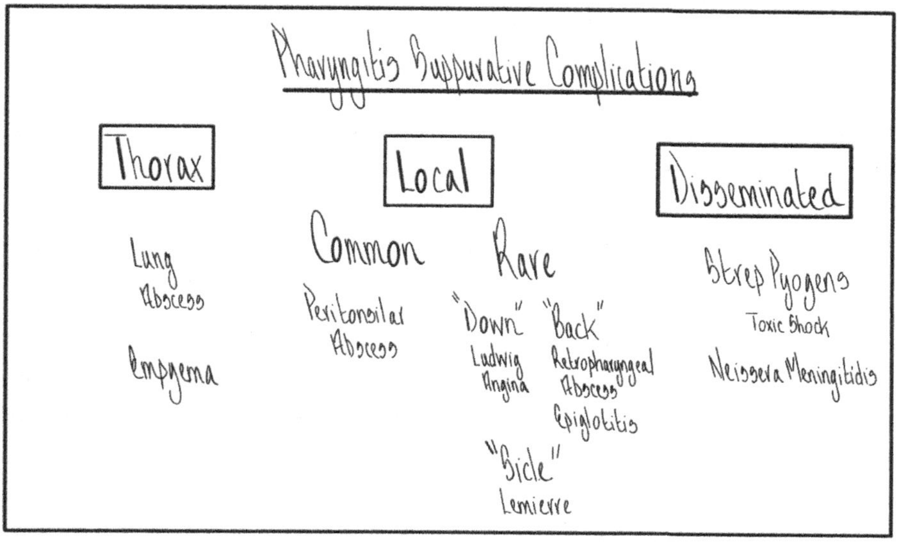

This figure organizes suppurative complications of pharyngitis based on how infection extends beyond the primary throat process. The central distinction is between contiguous local spread and hematogenous systemic dissemination.

Local complications reflect direct extension into adjacent anatomic spaces. Peritonsillar abscess represents the most common and typically localized form. In contrast, deeper infections extend along defined fascial planes and present with distinct patterns. Downward spread produces Ludwig's angina, a rapidly progressive infection of the submandibular and sublingual spaces marked by firm floor-of-mouth swelling, tongue elevation, and risk of airway compromise. Posterior extension leads to retropharyngeal abscess, involving the potential space behind the pharynx and associated with neck stiffness and airway risk. Epiglottitis represents adjacent airway involvement, characterized by rapid onset of sore throat, muffled voice, and drooling. Lateral spread results in

Lemierre syndrome, a septic thrombophlebitis of the internal jugular vein, often due to *Fusobacterium*, presenting with neck pain and septic emboli. Cervical necrotizing fasciitis reflects uncontrolled spread along fascial planes, with severe pain, tissue necrosis, systemic toxicity, and high mortality requiring urgent surgical management.

Disseminated complications arise from hematogenous spread. These include invasive *Streptococcus pyogenes* infection with potential toxic shock physiology, and invasive meningococcal disease, which may rapidly progress to sepsis, purpura, and multiorgan failure. In these cases, systemic instability often precedes or outweighs local throat findings.

The framework emphasizes a critical shift: progression beyond the tonsillar space—whether anatomically or systemically—signals increased risk. Once extension is suspected, the priority moves from routine testing to airway evaluation, imaging, and early specialty involvement.

Figure 2.1
Approach to unilateral leg erythema and swelling

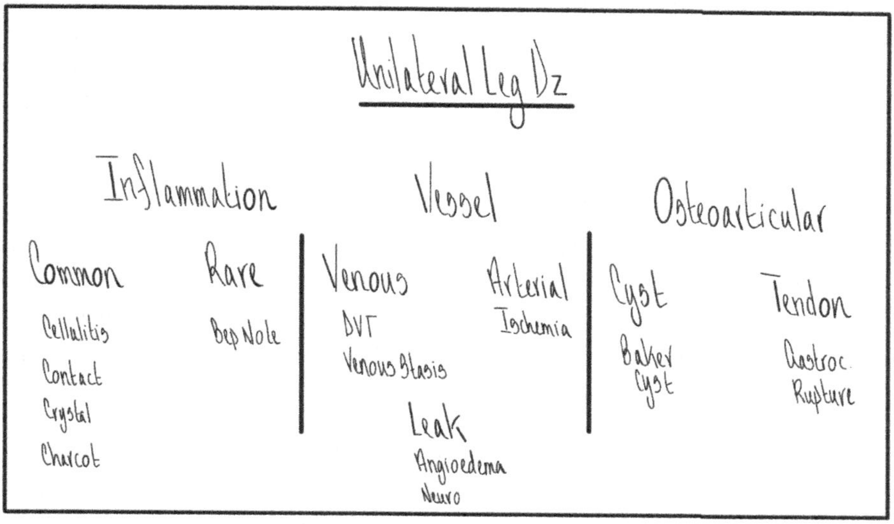

Not every red, swollen leg is cellulitis. Accurate evaluation begins by organizing the differential according to mechanism—distinguishing inflammatory, vascular, and osteoarticular processes before assigning a diagnosis.

Inflammatory causes reflect primary tissue or joint inflammation. Cellulitis presents with spreading erythema, warmth, and tenderness. Contact dermatitis produces localized redness following exposure to an irritant or allergen. Crystal disease, such as gout, is defined by abrupt-onset, intensely painful joint inflammation. Charcot arthropathy represents neuropathic joint destruction, often in diabetes, with warmth, swelling, and deformity that can mimic infection but occurs in the setting of reduced sensation.

Vascular causes reflect abnormalities in flow or vascular integrity. Venous processes include deep vein thrombosis, which presents with acute swelling and erythema, and chronic venous stasis, characterized by persistent, often bilateral redness without systemic signs of infection. Arterial insufficiency typically produces pain and pallor, though dependent rubor may be seen when the limb is lowered. Leak states include angioedema, marked by rapid, asymmetric swelling without warmth or tenderness, and neurogenic edema, in which chronic neuropathic changes produce non-infectious swelling and erythema that can resemble cellulitis but lack acute pain and systemic features.

Osteoarticular causes arise from structural injury or periarticular pathology. A ruptured Baker's cyst can cause sudden calf swelling and erythema, often with posterior knee fullness. Muscle or tendon injury, such as gastrocnemius rupture, presents with acute pain, swelling, and bruising following mechanical strain, with focal tenderness that distinguishes it from diffuse infection.

This framework emphasizes that similar-appearing presentations may arise from distinct mechanisms. Classifying by process—rather than appearance alone—reduces misdiagnosis and directs appropriate evaluation and management.

Figure 2.2
Cellulitis and gram-negative rods

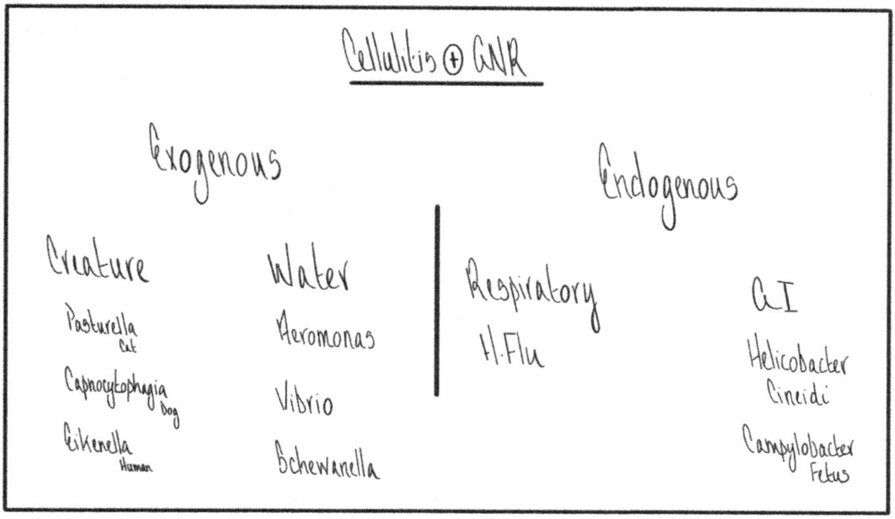

This figure organizes cellulitis in the setting of gram-negative bacteremia by distinguishing two mechanisms: exogenous inoculation and endogenous dissemination. Typical cellulitis arises from gram-positive skin flora through local extension after superficial injury. When gram-negative organisms are identified, the diagnostic frame must expand.

Exogenous sources reflect direct inoculation at the skin. Animal exposures—such as bites, scratches, or licks—can introduce organisms like *Pasteurella*. Environmental injuries, particularly involving water, may introduce *Vibrio*, *Aeromonas*, or *Shewanella* species. These exposures are not limited to classic aquatic settings; contaminated soil, brackish environments, and traumatic wounds can serve as entry points. In this pathway, infection begins at the skin and may subsequently progress to bloodstream involvement.

Endogenous sources reflect hematogenous spread from an internal reservoir. Organisms originating from the respiratory or gastrointestinal tract—such as *Haemophilus influenzae*, *Campylobacter fetus*, or *Helicobacter cinaedi*—can enter the bloodstream and seed peripheral tissues. In this branch, skin findings represent a secondary manifestation of systemic infection rather than the primary site.

This framework emphasizes a key diagnostic distinction: whether infection originates at the skin and spreads inward, or begins systemically and seeds the skin. Recognizing this directionality guides the search for exposures, underlying sources, and appropriate management.

Figure 3.1
Hemorrhage Overview: Open vs Closed Spaces

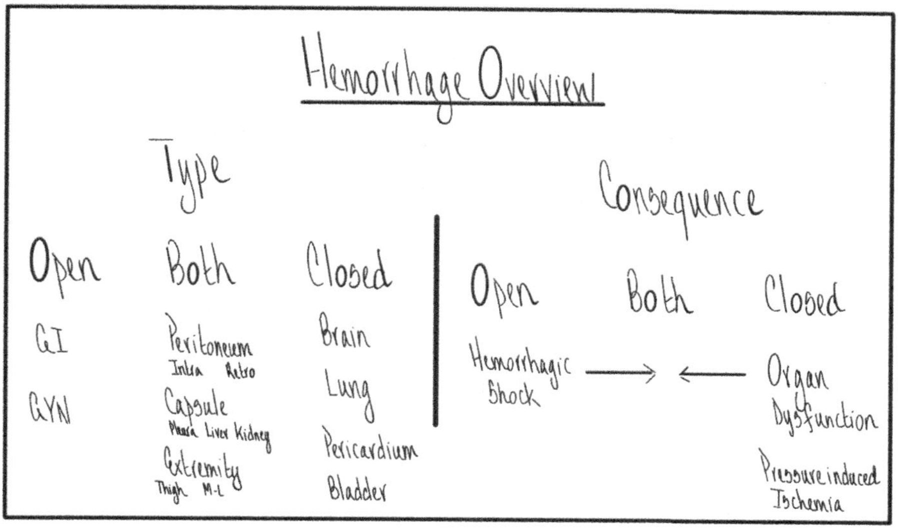

This figure organizes hemorrhage along two axes: anatomic containment (where the blood goes) and physiologic consequence (how that location causes harm).

The left half classifies bleeding by whether blood escapes into an open system or is confined within a closed compartment. Open systems, such as the gastrointestinal or genitourinary tract, typically present with visible blood loss and lead to hypovolemia and hemorrhagic shock. In contrast, closed spaces—including the cranial vault, thorax, pericardium, and bladder—limit external blood loss but produce organ dysfunction through local accumulation and pressure effects.

Some compartments behave along a spectrum. The peritoneum can accommodate large volumes of blood before clinical detection, functioning as a concealed reservoir. Organ capsules, such as those of the liver or kidney, may initially contain bleeding before rupture converts the process into a more extensive hemorrhage. Similarly, muscle and limb compartments—including the thigh—can sequester significant blood volume ("muscle-limb" compartments), leading to occult hypovolemia or local complications such as compartment syndrome.

The right half emphasizes consequence. Hemorrhage in open systems primarily results in hypovolemia and shock. In closed compartments, harm arises from pressure-induced ischemia: intracranial bleeding causes mass effect and herniation, pericardial bleeding impairs cardiac filling, and extremity bleeding may culminate in compartment syndrome.

This framework reinforces a core diagnostic move: when evaluating hemorrhage, ask where the blood is going and how that location produces injury. Location determines both urgency and mechanism.

Figure 3.2

Hematuria: An Anatomic Approach

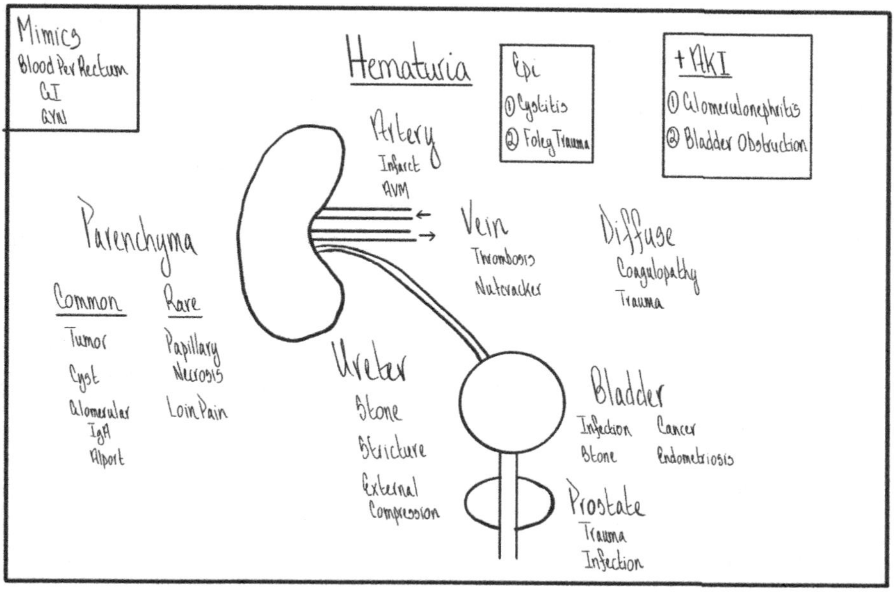

This figure organizes hematuria by anatomic source, emphasizing localization as the first diagnostic step. Rather than beginning with a list of causes, the framework moves sequentially along the urinary tract and its vascular supply, asking where blood enters the system.

The most common causes of hematuria include urinary tract infection, urolithiasis, and trauma, including from Foley catheterization.

Parenchymal causes arise from the kidney itself. Glomerular disease often produces dysmorphic red cells and proteinuria, reflecting a filtration barrier process. Structural lesions—such as tumors, cysts, or papillary necrosis—may present with pain or mass effect. Less common syndromes, including loin pain hematuria, fall within this category but are diagnoses of exclusion.

Vascular sources reflect abnormalities in blood flow. Arterial processes, such as infarction or arteriovenous malformation, typically present with abrupt onset and potential ischemic injury. Venous etiologies, including thrombosis or nutcracker syndrome, result from impaired outflow and elevated venous pressure. Distinguishing vascular from parenchymal disease guides both imaging strategy and urgency.

Downstream causes involve the collecting system and lower urinary tract. Ureteral pathology—most commonly stone or stricture—produces hematuria through mucosal irritation and obstruction, often with pain. Bladder sources include infection, malignancy, and stone. Prostatic bleeding may result from inflammation, instrumentation, or hypervascular tissue such as benign prostatic hyperplasia; however, because BPH is common and often coexists with other conditions, it should be considered a diagnosis of exclusion.

The framework is further shaped by clinical modifiers. Acute kidney injury raises concern for glomerular or obstructive processes. Severe pain suggests obstruction or infarction. Diffuse extra-renal bleeding points toward coagulopathy or systemic illness. Apparent hematuria may also reflect mimics, including menstrual, rectal, or cutaneous sources.

This approach reinforces a central principle: localize before labeling. Identifying where blood enters the urinary tract clarifies mechanism, prioritizes evaluation, and reduces premature closure.

Figure 4.1

Anorectal Pain: An Exam-Driven Framework

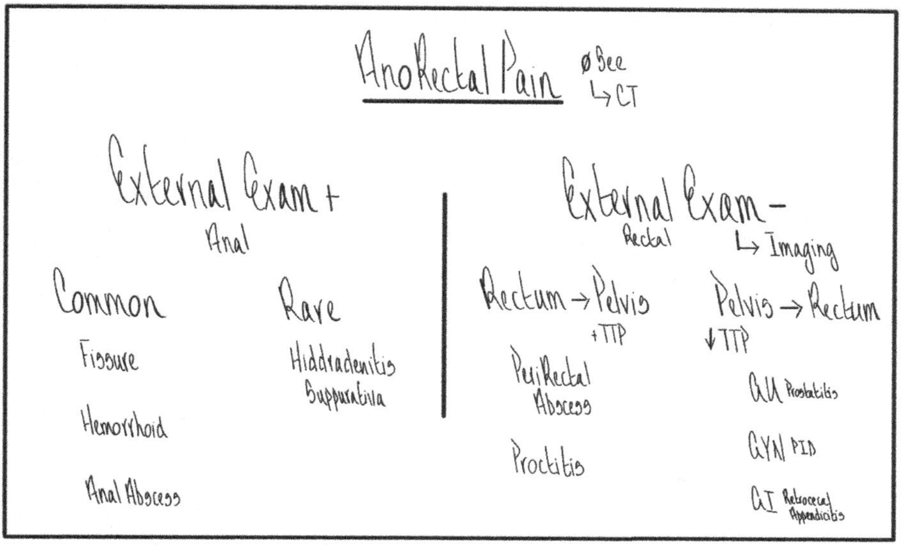

This figure organizes anorectal pain around a single pivot: the external examination. Evaluation begins with inspection and digital rectal examination, with localization preceding imaging.

When the external exam is positive, pathology is typically anal and directly accessible. Common causes include fissure, hemorrhoid, and superficial abscess. Less common conditions, such as hidradenitis suppurativa, arise from perianal skin and adnexal structures but follow the same principle of externally identifiable disease.

When the external exam is negative, the framework shifts inward. Pain may originate within the rectum and extend outward, as in perirectal abscess or proctitis, where digital rectal examination elicits significant tenderness. Alternatively, pain may arise from the pelvis and refer to the anorectal region, including genitourinary sources such as prostatitis, gynecologic conditions such as pelvic inflammatory disease, or gastrointestinal processes such as appendicitis. In these cases, rectal tenderness is often minimal or absent, reflecting a process outside the rectal wall.

When both external inspection and digital examination are unrevealing, imaging is typically required to identify deeper or referred sources of pain.

This framework emphasizes directionality: whether pain originates within the anorectal canal and extends outward, or arises from the pelvis and refers inward. Identifying this pattern guides evaluation and prevents premature reassurance when the exam is normal.

Figure 4.2

Rash + Proctitis: Infectious vs Autoimmune

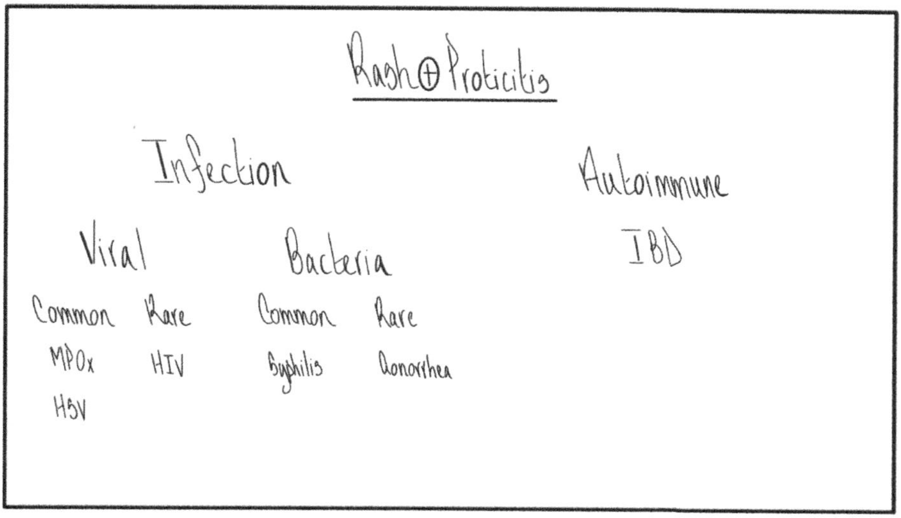

This figure organizes proctitis with rash into two mechanistic categories: infectious and immune-mediated. The central diagnostic task is determining whether inflammation reflects pathogen invasion or dysregulated immunity.

Infectious causes are most commonly sexually transmitted and often coexist due to shared modes of transmission and overlapping risk factors. Viral etiologies include herpes simplex virus and mpox. Bacterial pathogens include syphilis and gonorrhea. Human immunodeficiency virus may be present concurrently and can modify the clinical presentation. In this category, proctitis and rash represent manifestations of active infection, often involving multiple pathogens simultaneously.

When infectious causes are excluded or the presentation suggests chronic or relapsing disease, immune-mediated processes become more likely. Inflammatory bowel disease—particularly ulcerative colitis or Crohn disease involving the rectum—represents the primary consideration.

This framework emphasizes a key reasoning move: use mechanism to organize your thinking early. Distinguishing infection from immune-mediated disease helps prioritize and interpret testing, guides isolation precautions, and informs initial management.

Figure 5.1

Thrombosis Overview: Pump, Pipes, and Plasma

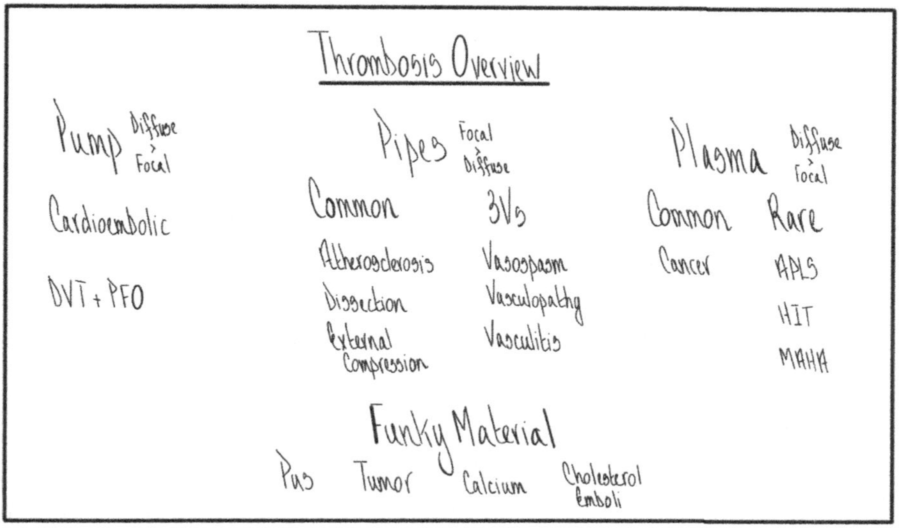

This figure organizes thrombosis into four mechanistic domains: abnormalities of the pump (heart), the pipe (vessels), the plasma (blood), and nonthrombotic intravascular material. The central task is identifying the source and mechanism of vascular occlusion.

Pump-mediated thrombosis reflects embolic events originating from the heart. Cardioembolic stroke and paradoxical embolism through a patent foramen ovale exemplify this mechanism, often producing sudden and multifocal vascular occlusions.

Pipe-mediated thrombosis arises from pathology within the vessel itself. Atherosclerosis, arterial dissection, and external compression create localized endothelial injury and flow disturbance. Less common causes include vasculitis, vasculopathy, and vasospasm. These processes typically produce territorial or organ-specific ischemia.

Plasma-mediated thrombosis reflects systemic hypercoagulability. Malignancy-associated thrombosis is among the most common causes, along with heparin-induced thrombocytopenia and microangiopathic processes. These conditions predispose to recurrent or multifocal thrombosis across vascular beds.

A key distinction lies in distribution: pump and plasma disorders tend to produce diffuse or multifocal events, whereas pipe disease usually affects a single vascular territory.

Finally, some occlusions result from nonthrombotic intravascular material, including tumor emboli, septic emboli, cholesterol emboli, or particulate debris, emphasizing that not all vascular obstruction represents true thrombus.

This framework reinforces a central principle: use mechanism to structure your approach. Considering pump, pipe, plasma, or material helps organize testing and guide early management, even as multiple possibilities are evaluated in parallel.

Figure 5.2
Dialysis Access Complications: A Mechanistic Overview

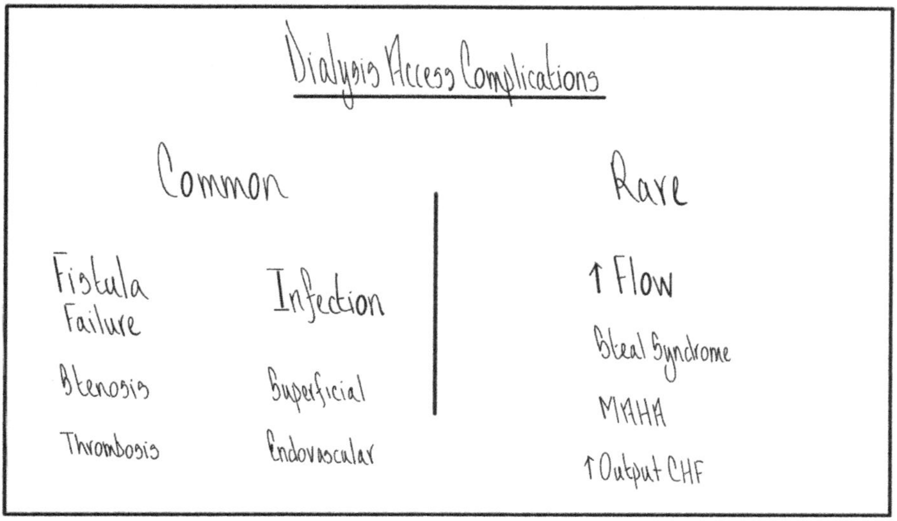

This figure organizes complications of arteriovenous fistula for dialysis access into common and flow-related mechanisms.

The most common complications are fistula failure and infection. Failure is typically due to outflow stenosis, with or without superimposed thrombosis, leading to inadequate dialysis. Infection may involve the overlying skin or extend into the vascular system, where it can result in bacteremia and systemic illness.

A distinct and clinically important category involves excessive flow through the fistula. High-flow states can divert blood away from the distal limb, resulting in dialysis-associated steal syndrome with ischemic pain. Turbulent flow may produce shear stress and lead to microangiopathic hemolytic anemia. In severe cases, increased venous return can overwhelm cardiac capacity and result in high-output heart failure.

This framework emphasizes mechanism: whether complications arise from obstruction, infection, or excessive flow. Identifying the underlying process guides evaluation and management.

Figure 6.1

Polyuria: Solute versus Solvent Framework

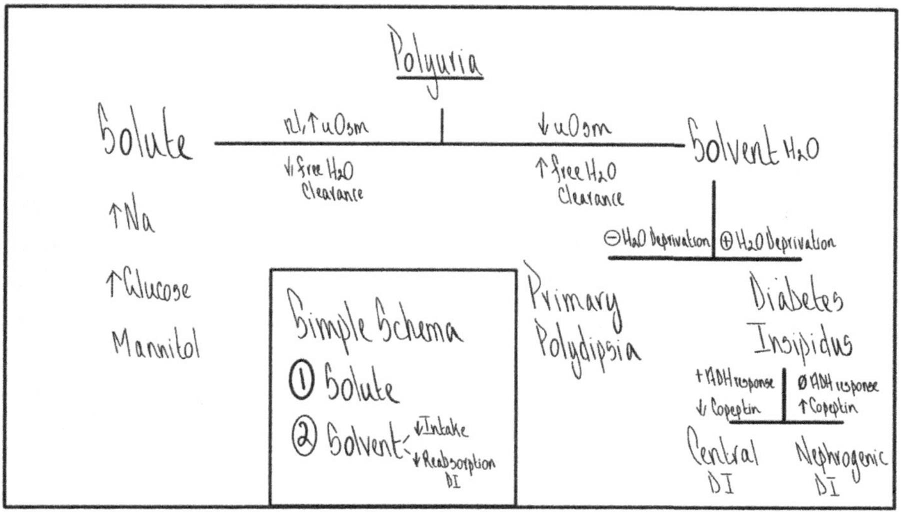

Evaluation of polyuria begins with a key branch point: urine osmolality. This can be quickly estimated from urine specific gravity using the approximation "last two digits × 30" (e.g., 1.010 ≈ 300 mOsm/kg). Urine osmolality determines whether excess urine output is driven by solute or water.

Normal or elevated urine osmolality indicates solute diuresis. In this setting, the kidneys excrete osmotically active particles that obligate water loss. Common causes include hyperglycemia, increased sodium load, or osmotic agents such as mannitol.

Low urine osmolality indicates water (solvent) diuresis. Here, the urine is dilute, reflecting high free water clearance due to impaired water reabsorption. This occurs with excessive water intake (primary polydipsia) or defects in vasopressin secretion or renal response (diabetes insipidus).

When water diuresis is identified, further distinction relies on physiologic testing. During water deprivation, intact vasopressin function leads to urine concentration, consistent with primary polydipsia. Failure to concentrate urine indicates diabetes insipidus, which may be central (impaired vasopressin secretion) or nephrogenic (renal resistance to vasopressin).

This framework emphasizes a central diagnostic move: determine whether polyuria is driven by solute or water. Concentrated urine (normal or high osmolality) indicates solute diuresis, whereas dilute urine (low osmolality) reflects water diuresis, prompting evaluation for primary polydipsia or diabetes insipidus. This distinction localizes physiology, guides testing, and directs management.

Figure 6.2

Central and Nephrogenic Diabetes Insipidus

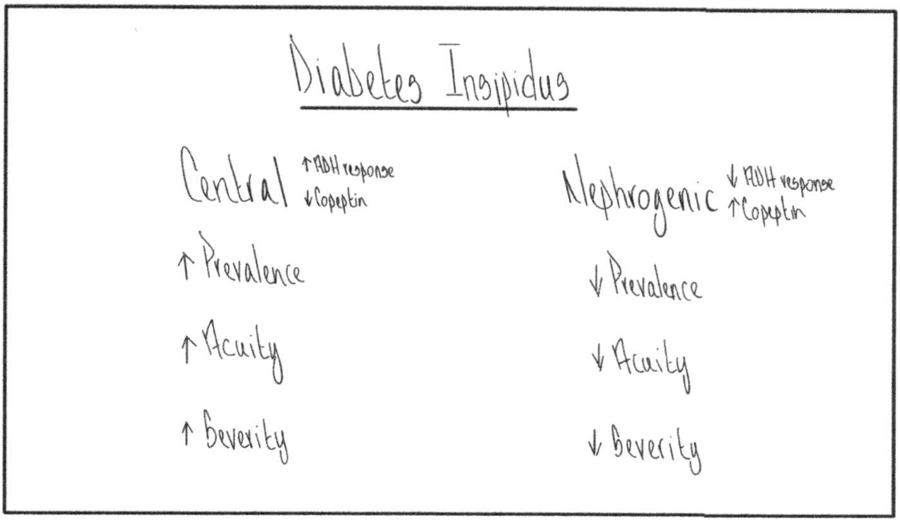

This figure organizes diabetes insipidus by physiologic localization: impaired vasopressin secretion versus renal resistance to vasopressin. The central diagnostic task is to determine whether the defect lies in hormone production or in the kidney's ability to respond.

Central diabetes insipidus results from reduced vasopressin secretion from the posterior pituitary. Copeptin, a surrogate marker of vasopressin, is typically low and supports the diagnosis. Urine concentration improves after administration of desmopressin, reflecting intact renal responsiveness.

Nephrogenic diabetes insipidus arises from renal resistance to vasopressin. In this setting, copeptin levels are typically elevated, indicating preserved hormone production. Despite desmopressin administration, the urine remains dilute, confirming a defect at the level of the kidney.

Clinically, central diabetes insipidus often presents more acutely, whereas nephrogenic disease tends to develop gradually unless triggered by medications or metabolic disturbances.

This framework emphasizes physiologic localization. Distinguishing impaired secretion from impaired renal response directs diagnostic testing and determines appropriate management.

Figure 7.1
Portal Vein Thrombosis: Etiologic Categories

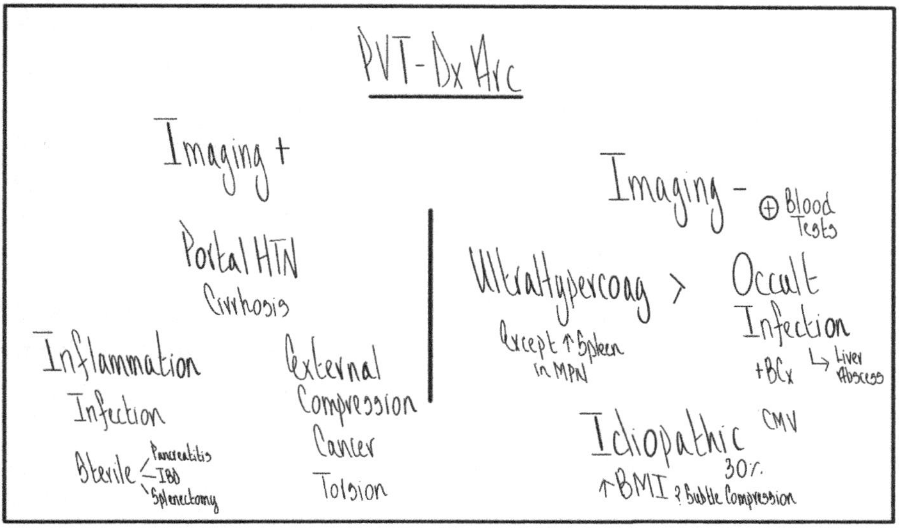

This figure organizes portal vein thrombosis by a key diagnostic distinction: imaging-positive versus imaging-negative etiologies. While cirrhosis remains the most common cause—through portal hypertension, sluggish flow, and a prothrombotic state—the evaluation requires identifying whether a local precipitant is visible.

Imaging-positive etiologies reflect local factors affecting the portal system. Cirrhosis is often evident through architectural changes and altered portal flow. Intra-abdominal inflammation, including appendicitis, diverticulitis, cholecystitis, or pancreatitis, can promote thrombosis through local injury and stasis. Noninfectious conditions such as inflammatory bowel disease or prior splenectomy may contribute similarly. External compression from malignancy—particularly pancreatic, hepatic, or biliary tumors—or mechanical distortion of the portal vein represents another important category.

Imaging-negative etiologies reflect systemic or occult processes. Hypercoagulable states are among the most common, especially myeloproliferative neoplasms associated with JAK2 mutations, where splenomegaly may be the only imaging clue. Occult infection should be considered when blood cultures are positive without a clear source, particularly from gastrointestinal origins; organisms such as *Fusobacterium nucleatum* can be implicated in this context. Subtle or missed infections, including liver abscess or cytomegalovirus, may also contribute. A substantial proportion of cases remain idiopathic, with elevated body mass index recognized as a risk factor.

This framework emphasizes a central diagnostic move: determine whether portal vein thrombosis is driven by a local, imaging-visible process or by a systemic or occult condition. This distinction guides further evaluation and management.

Figure 7.2

Hepatic Infection: Localizing Parenchyma Versus Plumbing

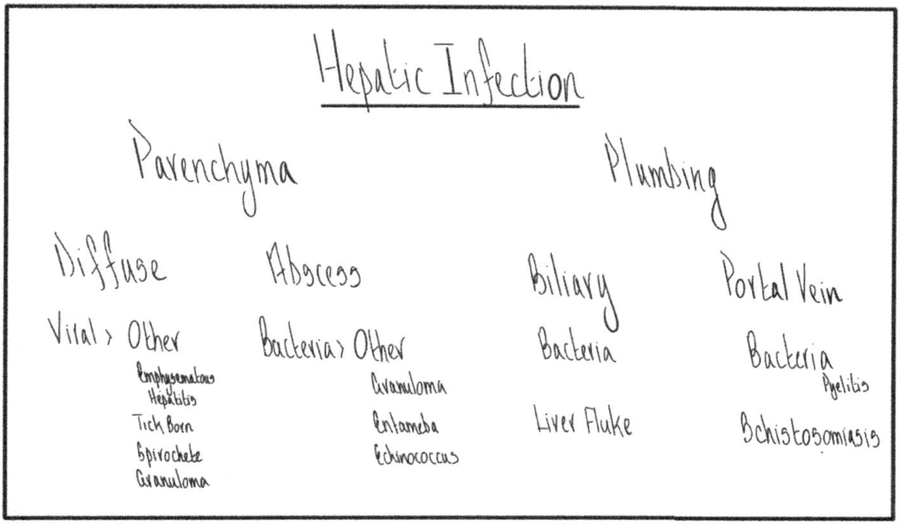

This figure organizes hepatic infection using a compartment-based framework: parenchymal disease involving the liver tissue itself, and infection of the hepatic "plumbing," including the biliary and vascular systems. The central task is to localize the process before identifying the pathogen.

Parenchymal infections may be diffuse or focal. Diffuse involvement is most commonly viral. Other causes include granulomatous and atypical infections—such as tuberculosis, histoplasmosis, or brucellosis—as well as less common systemic infections like ehrlichiosis or leptospirosis. Rare entities, such as emphysematous hepatitis, represent severe bacterial infection with gas formation within the liver.

Focal parenchymal disease most often reflects abscess formation in this context. Bacterial abscesses are commonly caused by enteric organisms such as *Escherichia coli*, *Klebsiella*, and streptococcal species. Parasitic infections, including *Entamoeba histolytica* and *Echinococcus*, produce characteristic focal lesions such as amebic abscesses or hydatid cysts. Granulomatous infections may also present as focal hepatic lesions.

Infections of the hepatic "plumbing" arise within the biliary or portal venous systems. Acute cholangitis results from biliary obstruction with ascending infection, commonly involving enteric bacteria. Portal venous infection (pylephlebitis) reflects septic thrombophlebitis, often originating from intra-abdominal inflammation and involving anaerobic organisms. Parasitic infections such as schistosomiasis can affect the portal system and lead to chronic hepatic complications.

The distribution of hepatic infection varies with geography, exposure, and host factors, with parasitic and granulomatous diseases more common in endemic regions.

This framework emphasizes localization as the first diagnostic step: determine whether infection involves the liver parenchyma or its vascular and biliary systems. This distinction clarifies pathogenesis, guides evaluation, and directs management.

Figure 8.1
Persistent Pulmonary Opacity: Pneumonia Mimics

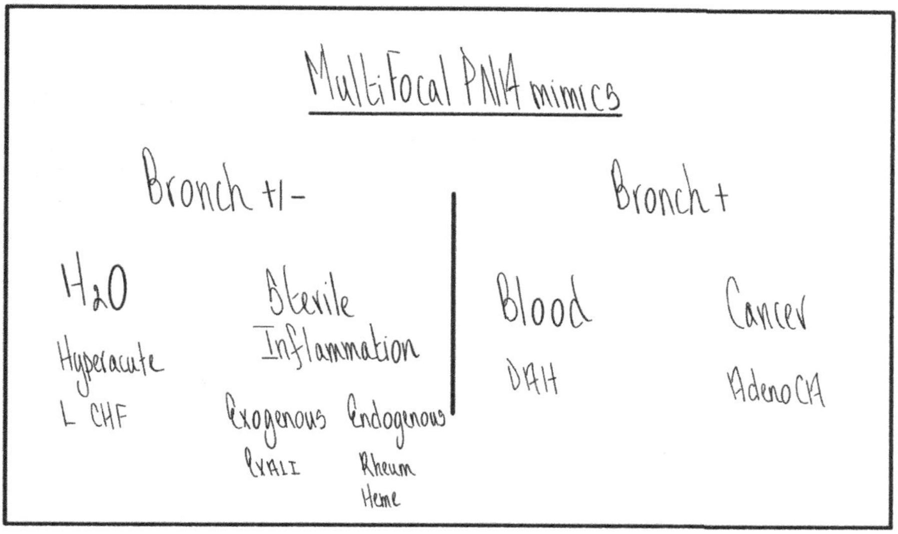

This figure organizes persistent pulmonary opacity using a mechanistic framework. When radiographic findings fail to resolve, the diagnostic task shifts from empiric antibiotic escalation to identifying the underlying process.

Infectious causes, including atypical, mycobacterial, fungal, or indolent pathogens, remain important considerations. However, lack of response to appropriate therapy should prompt evaluation for noninfectious etiologies, often with bronchoscopy as a key diagnostic tool.

Bronchoscopy provides a critical branch point. A positive examination may reveal blood in the airways, indicating diffuse alveolar hemorrhage, or malignant cells, suggesting an underlying neoplastic process. These findings localize pathology to the alveolar space or airway.

A negative bronchoscopy suggests alternative mechanisms. Cardiogenic processes, such as acute left-sided heart failure, can produce alveolar flooding without airway pathology. Noninfectious inflammatory conditions—including inhalational injury (e.g., EVALI), autoimmune disease, or hematologic disorders—may also present with persistent opacities despite sterile airways.

This framework emphasizes a central diagnostic shift: from treating presumed infection to identifying mechanism. Asking what process is filling the alveoli—blood, fluid, cells, or inflammation—guides further evaluation and management.

Figure 8.2
Granuloma: Mechanistic Differential

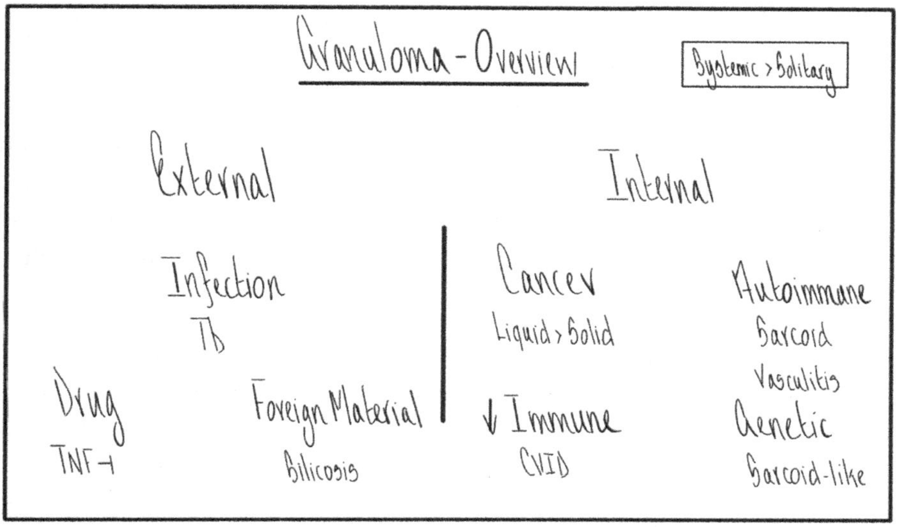

Granulomatous inflammation represents a structured immune response to persistent stimuli and is best approached through a mechanistic framework that distinguishes external (exogenous) from internal (endogenous) drivers.

External causes reflect the immune system's attempt to contain foreign material or organisms, most commonly infection. Mycobacterial disease, particularly tuberculosis, is the classic example, while fungal pathogens such as *Histoplasma* or *Cryptococcus* can produce similar responses. Other infections, including non-tuberculous mycobacteria and select bacterial pathogens, should be considered based on exposure and geography. Noninfectious external triggers include drugs—especially tumor necrosis factor inhibitors—and foreign materials such as silica, beryllium, talc, or silicone, which provoke granuloma formation through chronic immune activation.

Internal causes arise from dysregulated host biology rather than an external inciting agent. Immune-mediated and inflammatory conditions form a major category, with sarcoidosis as the prototypical noninfectious granulomatous disease. Vasculitic disorders, such as granulomatosis with polyangiitis, and chronic inflammatory conditions, including Crohn's disease, may also produce granulomas. Immune deficiency states, such as common variable immunodeficiency, can present with widespread granulomatous involvement reflecting impaired immune regulation. Malignancy, particularly hematologic cancers such as lymphoma, may provoke granulomatous responses that obscure or accompany the underlying disease.

A key diagnostic principle is that granulomas are a reaction pattern, not a diagnosis. While infection remains the most common cause, noninfectious etiologies are frequent and often mimic one another. Non-caseating granulomas do not establish sarcoidosis; evaluation requires exclusion of infection and malignancy, followed by integration of clinical context, exposures, and systemic findings.

This framework emphasizes a central reasoning move: identify whether the granulomatous response reflects an external exposure or an internal dysregulated process to guide diagnosis and management.

Figure 9.1
Lymphocytosis: Polyclonal vs. Monoclonal

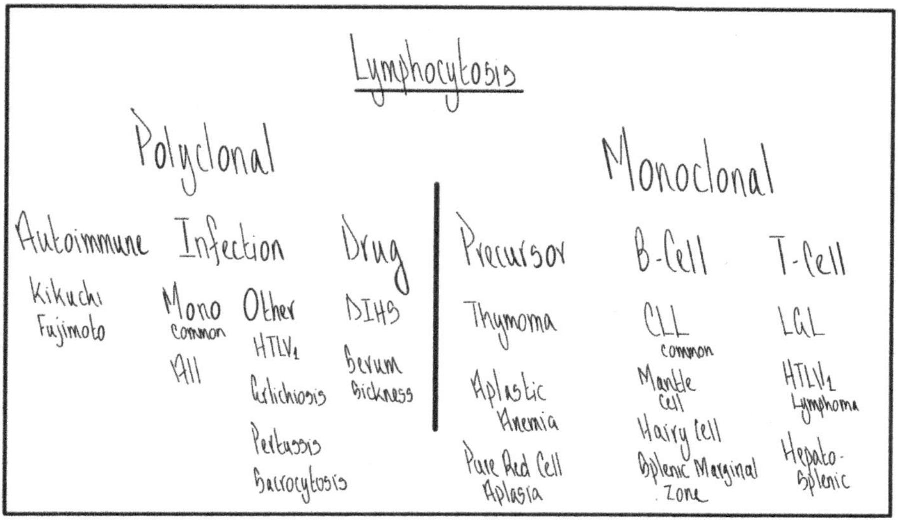

Lymphocytosis is defined by an increased absolute lymphocyte count and is best classified by clonality into polyclonal (reactive) and monoclonal (neoplastic) forms. The central diagnostic task is to determine whether lymphocyte expansion reflects a reactive immune response or a neoplastic process.

Polyclonal lymphocytosis is far more common and typically arises from infection or immune activation. Viral infections are the predominant cause, including mononucleosis syndromes due to Epstein–Barr virus, cytomegalovirus, or human immunodeficiency virus. Bacterial and atypical infections, such as pertussis or tick-borne illnesses, may also produce lymphocytosis. Drug reactions and immune-mediated conditions, including drug hypersensitivity syndromes and autoimmune disease, represent additional causes. In these settings, the lymphocyte population is heterogeneous, reflecting a reactive process.

Monoclonal lymphocytosis results from clonal expansion of B or T lymphocytes and suggests an underlying lymphoproliferative disorder. Chronic lymphocytic leukemia is the most common cause in adults. Other B-cell and T-cell neoplasms, including large granular lymphocyte leukemia, may present similarly. These conditions are often persistent and may be associated with cytopenias, lymphadenopathy, or splenomegaly.

Clinical features help guide suspicion. Transient lymphocytosis in a younger patient favors a reactive process, whereas persistent lymphocytosis, especially in older adults or in the presence of cytopenias or organomegaly, raises concern for clonality. Flow cytometry is the key diagnostic test to distinguish polyclonal from monoclonal populations.

This framework emphasizes a central principle: determine clonality before labeling the cause. Identifying whether lymphocytosis is reactive or clonal directs evaluation, prognosis, and management.

Figure 9.2

Persistent Hiccups: Localizing Along the Reflex Arc

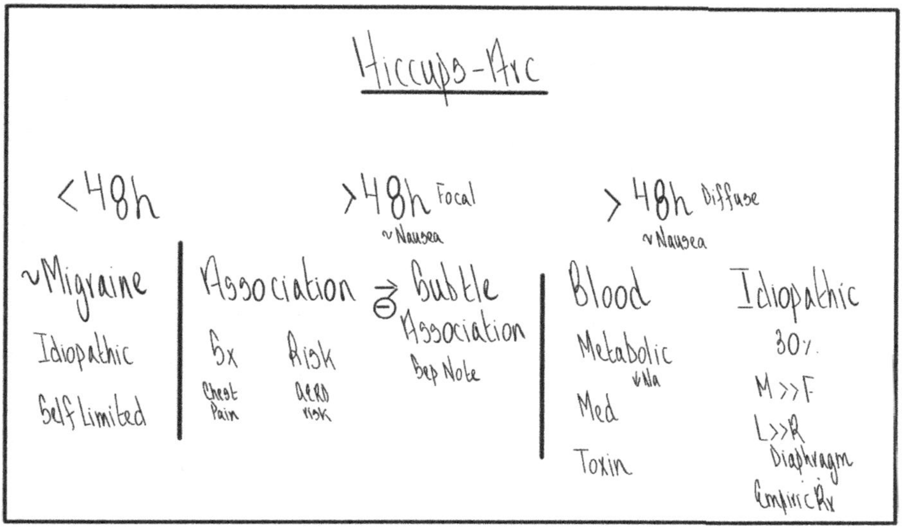

This figure organizes the evaluation of hiccups using a familiar diagnostic approach: duration as the initial branch point, followed by symptom-based localization. As with migraine and nausea, the key task is determining when to shift from reassurance to targeted evaluation.

Hiccups lasting less than 48 hours are most often transient and benign. Common triggers include gastric distension, alcohol, and carbonated beverages. These brief episodes reflect temporary diaphragmatic irritation and typically resolve with reassurance and simple maneuvers such as breath holding or cold water ingestion.

When hiccups persist beyond 48 hours, the diagnostic approach shifts toward localization. Associated symptoms help identify the source of irritation along the hiccup reflex arc. Thoracic processes (e.g., pneumonia or pericardial disease), abdominal pathology (e.g., hepatobiliary or subdiaphragmatic disease), and central nervous system lesions should be considered based on the clinical context. Subtle symptoms, such as reflux, may require careful elicitation.

In the absence of localizing features, metabolic and toxic causes should be evaluated. Electrolyte disturbances, uremia, and medication effects can lower the threshold for reflex activation and produce persistent hiccups.

Many cases remain idiopathic despite evaluation, particularly in older individuals. The critical inflection point is duration: transient hiccups are managed symptomatically, whereas persistent hiccups require anatomical and mechanistic localization.

Figure 10

Hyperglycemia: Organizing Acute and End-Organ Complications

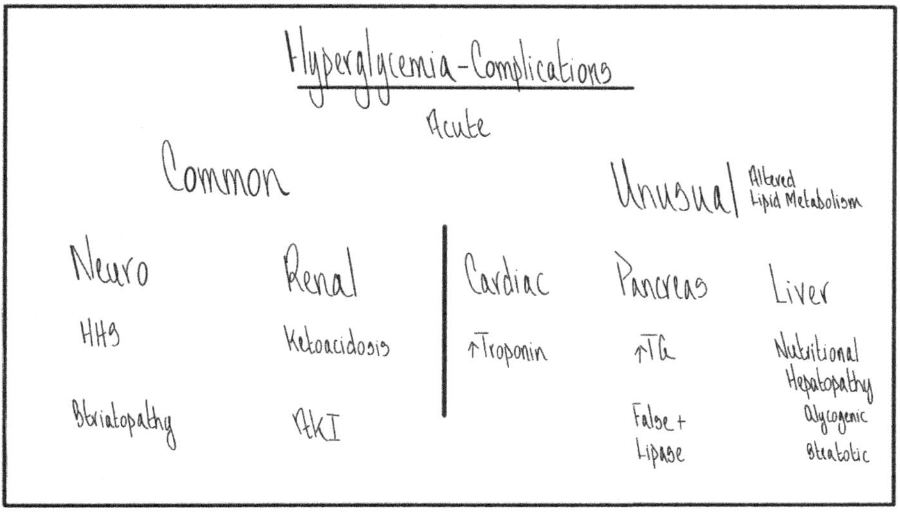

This figure organizes hyperglycemia by patterns of acute end-organ injury rather than glucose level alone, emphasizing that its clinical significance lies in its systemic effects.

Acute metabolic emergencies such as diabetic ketoacidosis and hyperosmolar hyperglycemic state reflect profound insulin deficiency and dehydration, leading to osmotic diuresis, electrolyte disturbances, and altered mental status. Neurologic complications are common, ranging from global encephalopathy in hyperosmolar states to focal syndromes such as hyperglycemic striatopathy.

Renal involvement is frequent. Volume depletion from osmotic diuresis reduces renal perfusion and may result in acute kidney injury, initially prerenal and potentially progressing to intrinsic injury if uncorrected.

Cardiac injury during severe hyperglycemia is often due to demand ischemia, with troponin elevation reflecting metabolic stress rather than acute coronary occlusion.

Metabolic consequences may involve other organs. Hypertriglyceridemia can precipitate pancreatitis, though interpretation may be confounded by enzyme elevations in ketoacidosis. Hepatic manifestations, including steatosis and glycogenic hepatopathy, reflect substrate excess and altered metabolic regulation.

This framework emphasizes a central principle: hyperglycemia is a marker of systemic metabolic stress rather than an isolated laboratory abnormality. Recognizing patterns of organ involvement—neurologic, renal, cardiac, and metabolic—guides evaluation and management beyond the glucose value itself.

Figure 11.1

Symptomatic Bradycardia: Targeted and Empiric Treatment

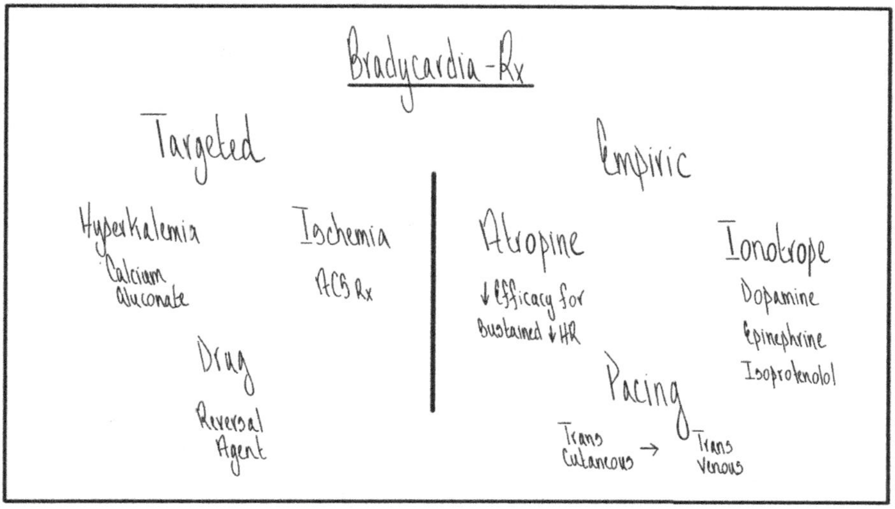

This figure organizes management of symptomatic bradycardia into two parallel priorities: targeted treatment of the underlying cause and empiric hemodynamic support. The first question is not the etiology but perfusion. Hypotension, altered mental status, ischemic chest discomfort, or signs of shock require urgent intervention.

Targeted therapy addresses reversible causes. In hyperkalemia, intravenous calcium is administered to stabilize the cardiac membrane, followed by therapies that shift potassium intracellularly or enhance its elimination. When bradycardia is due to myocardial ischemia, rapid reperfusion is the priority. In drug-induced cases, the offending agent should be discontinued and, when available, specific reversal agents administered.

Empiric therapy supports perfusion while the cause is identified. Atropine is first-line for vagally mediated bradycardia but may be ineffective in intrinsic conduction disease. If instability persists, chronotropic infusions such as dopamine or epinephrine can provide temporary support. When pharmacologic therapy is insufficient or structural conduction disease is present, pacing is required, typically beginning with transcutaneous pacing and escalating to transvenous pacing if needed.

In practice, empiric support and targeted therapy proceed in parallel to stabilize the patient while addressing the underlying mechanism. Permanent pacing may be required when reversible causes are excluded.

This framework emphasizes a central principle: stabilize first, localize second, and correct the trigger. A slow heart rate is a number; symptomatic bradycardia is a problem of perfusion.

Figure 11.2

Acute Bradycardia: Extrinsic vs. Intrinsic Causes

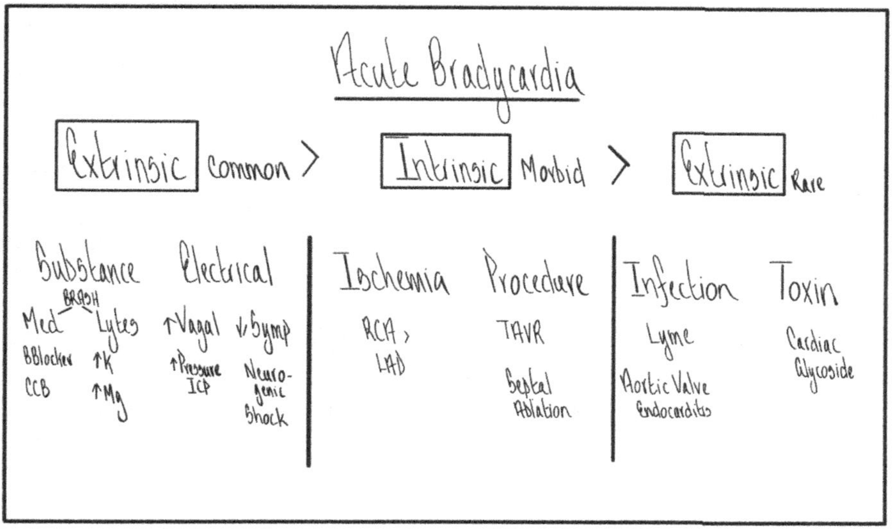

This figure categorizes acute bradycardia by mechanism, distinguishing between extrinsic causes and intrinsic disease of the conduction system. The central diagnostic task is to determine whether the sinus node is functionally suppressed or structurally impaired.

Extrinsic causes are most common and often reversible. Medications—particularly beta-blockers and non-dihydropyridine calcium channel blockers—depress sinus node activity and atrioventricular conduction. Electrolyte disturbances, especially hyperkalemia, disrupt cardiac depolarization and can produce significant bradycardia; BRASH syndrome represents a convergence of renal failure, AV nodal blockade, and hyperkalemia leading to profound instability. Autonomic influences are also important: increased vagal tone, decreased sympathetic output, or reflex-mediated responses (e.g., from intracranial or visceral stimuli) can transiently suppress heart rate.

Intrinsic causes reflect structural or ischemic injury to the conduction system and are typically more persistent. Acute coronary ischemia, particularly involving the right coronary artery, commonly affects the sinoatrial and atrioventricular nodes. Procedural injury, such as after transcatheter aortic valve replacement or septal interventions, may also disrupt conduction pathways.

Less common extrinsic causes include autonomic disorders, infections, and toxins. Conditions such as Lyme disease or endocarditis may involve the conduction system, while agents like digoxin or other toxins can impair nodal function through pharmacologic effects.

This framework emphasizes a central principle: localize the mechanism before escalating therapy. Distinguishing extrinsic suppression from intrinsic conduction disease guides both evaluation and management.

Figure 12.1
Constipation: Red Flags That Warrant Imaging or Further Evaluation

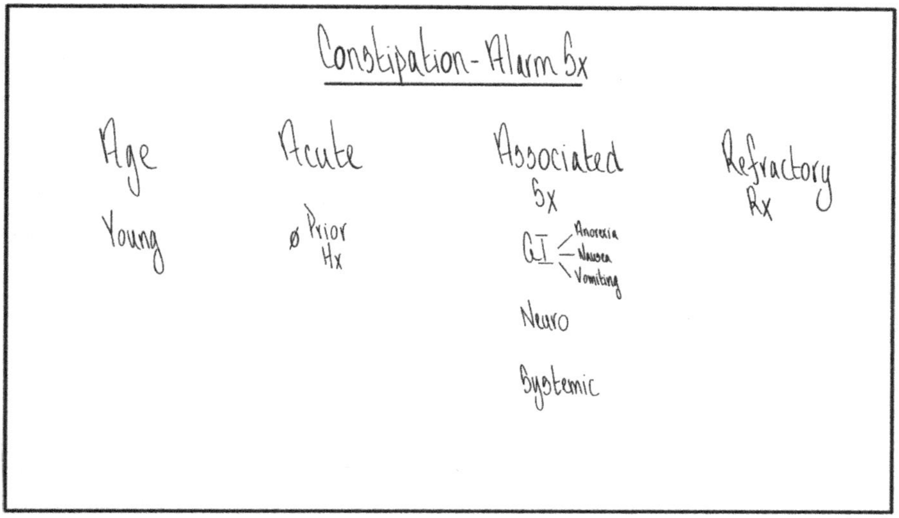

This figure organizes constipation by risk pattern rather than symptom alone. Most cases are benign, often related to decreased fluid intake, low fiber, inactivity, or idiopathic causes. The diagnostic task is to identify features that suggest a more serious underlying process.

Concerning patterns emerge from associated symptoms. Acute onset or progressive symptoms, particularly when accompanied by nausea, vomiting, or significant abdominal pain, raise concern for obstruction or ileus. Neurologic features—such as lower extremity weakness, gait disturbance, saddle anesthesia, or urinary retention—suggest spinal cord or autonomic dysfunction rather than primary gastrointestinal disease. Systemic findings, including anemia, weight loss, or constitutional symptoms, point toward inflammatory or malignant etiologies.

Response to therapy is also informative. Constipation that persists despite appropriate treatment should prompt reassessment, as refractory symptoms may signal an unrecognized structural or systemic cause.

This framework emphasizes pattern recognition over reflex treatment. Constipation is common; dangerous constipation reveals itself through context.

Figure 12.2
Neurologic Dysfunction with Urinary Retention: Localization Framework

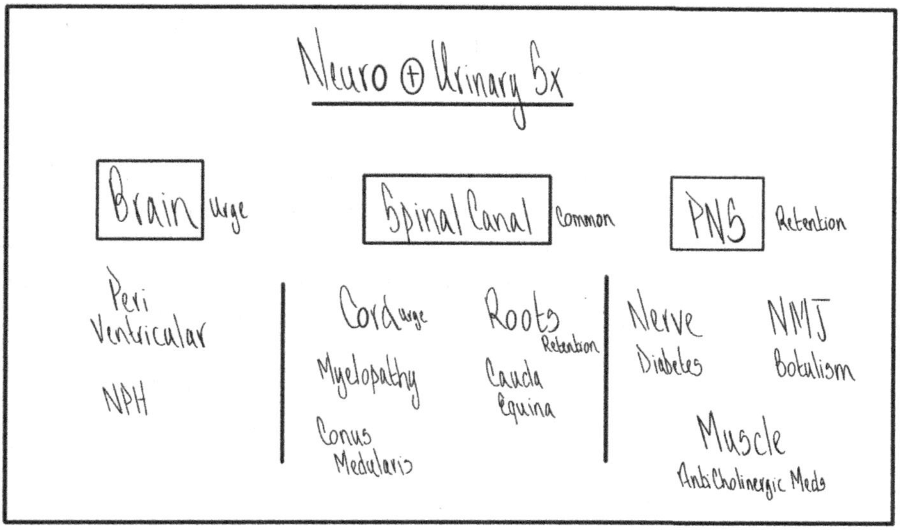

This figure localizes urinary retention in the presence of neurologic symptoms along the neuroaxis, emphasizing that the pattern of bladder dysfunction helps identify the level of involvement. Brain lesions, particularly periventricular processes such as normal pressure hydrocephalus, typically produce urge incontinence rather than true urinary retention, reflecting loss of central inhibitory control.

Spinal pathology requires further distinction. Cord lesions, including myelopathy or conus medullaris involvement, more often present with urgency or incontinence due to disruption of descending control. In contrast, root-level pathology—classically in cauda equina syndrome—leads to urinary retention, often preceding overt motor weakness and serving as a key localizing feature.

Peripheral causes reflect impaired bladder contraction or autonomic dysfunction. Advanced autonomic neuropathy, most commonly due to diabetes, can result in incomplete emptying and retention. Medication effects are a frequent and often reversible cause, particularly from anticholinergic agents and opioids. Less common contributors include peripheral nerve and neuromuscular junction disorders, such as botulism. Guillain–Barré syndrome may involve autonomic dysfunction but often spares bladder function early in its course.

This framework emphasizes a central diagnostic move: when urinary retention accompanies neurologic symptoms, prioritize localization. Retention shifts concern toward root or peripheral involvement, whereas urgency or incontinence more often reflects suprasacral or central processes. Early recognition of these patterns is critical, as conditions such as cauda equina syndrome require urgent evaluation and intervention.

Figure 13.1
Photophobia: Anatomic Localization Framework

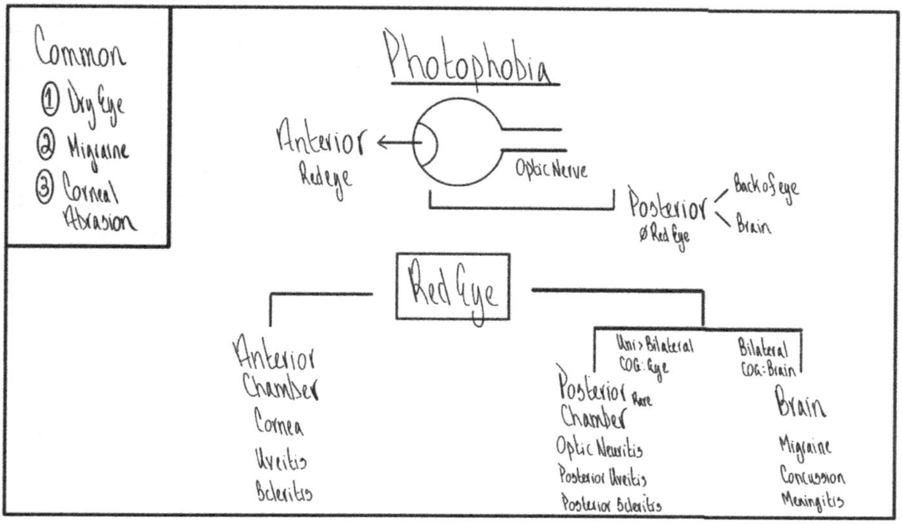

This figure organizes photophobia by anatomic localization, distinguishing anterior segment disease from posterior or central processes. The central diagnostic task is to determine whether light sensitivity arises from ocular surface inflammation or from deeper or intracranial pathology.

Common causes include dry eye, migraine, and corneal abrasion. Dry eye and corneal abrasion produce photophobia through disruption of the corneal surface and exposure of sensory nerve endings, typically resulting in unilateral discomfort. Migraine, by contrast, reflects central sensory dysregulation and often presents with bilateral light sensitivity.

The presence or absence of eye redness provides a key branch point. A red eye suggests anterior segment pathology. Corneal processes, such as abrasion or surface irritation, cause acute pain and photophobia. Uveitis presents with ciliary injection, pain, and light sensitivity, often with consensual photophobia. Scleritis produces deeper, more severe pain and may be associated with systemic autoimmune disease.

A quiet eye shifts the focus to posterior or central causes. Posterior ocular processes, such as optic neuritis or posterior uveitis, are less common and often unilateral, typically accompanied by visual changes. In contrast, central nervous system causes—including migraine, meningitis, concussion, or subarachnoid hemorrhage—are usually bilateral and associated with systemic or neurologic symptoms.

This framework emphasizes localization through a simple clinical pivot: red eye versus quiet eye. Integrating laterality and associated findings clarifies the source of photophobia and guides further evaluation.

Figure 13.2
Headache: Clinical Features That Raise Concern for Secondary Causes

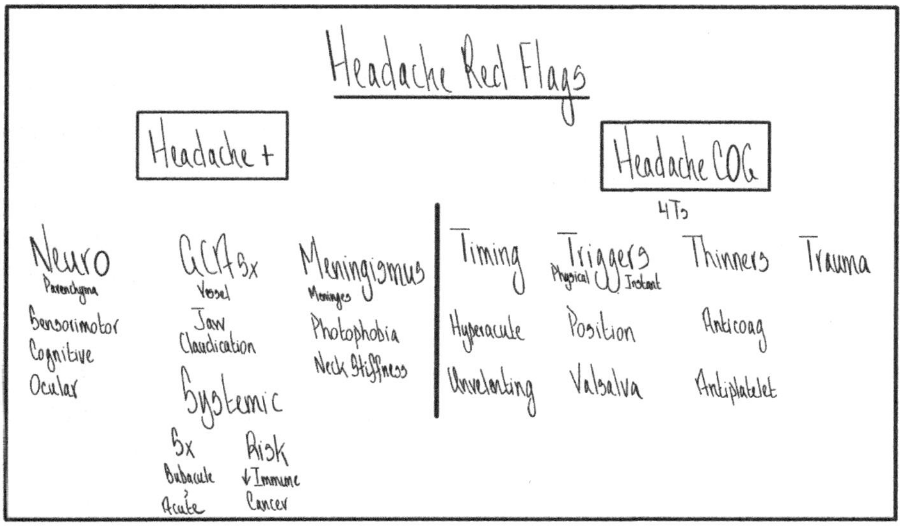

Most headaches encountered in clinical practice are primary and not due to an underlying structural or systemic disease. The diagnostic task is to identify features that suggest a secondary cause.

Secondary headache should be considered when the presentation deviates from a patient's baseline or when red flag features are present. These features fall into two groups: localizing symptoms and high-risk patterns summarized by the "4 Ts."

Localizing symptoms suggest involvement of specific structures. New focal neurologic deficits, altered cognition, or visual disturbances raise concern for parenchymal disease such as stroke, hemorrhage, or encephalitis. In patients over 50, headache with jaw claudication, scalp tenderness, or visual symptoms suggests giant cell arteritis. Headache accompanied by fever, neck stiffness, or photophobia points toward meningitis. Subacute or progressive headache with systemic features—such as weight loss, fever, or immunocompromise—raises concern for infection, malignancy, or inflammatory disease.

The "4 Ts" identify high-risk patterns. Timing refers to sudden-onset or rapidly progressive headache, concerning for vascular events such as subarachnoid hemorrhage. Triggers include Valsalva, exertion, or positional changes, suggesting altered intracranial pressure or structural lesions. Thinners (anticoagulant or antiplatelet use) increase the risk of intracranial bleeding, even with minimal provocation. Trauma, particularly in older adults or those with bleeding risk, raises concern for subdural hematoma.

This framework emphasizes structured risk assessment. Red flag features are cumulative, and the goal is not indiscriminate testing but thoughtful adjustment of diagnostic probability based on pattern, associated symptoms, and patient context.

Figure 14.1
Acute liver disease: localize first

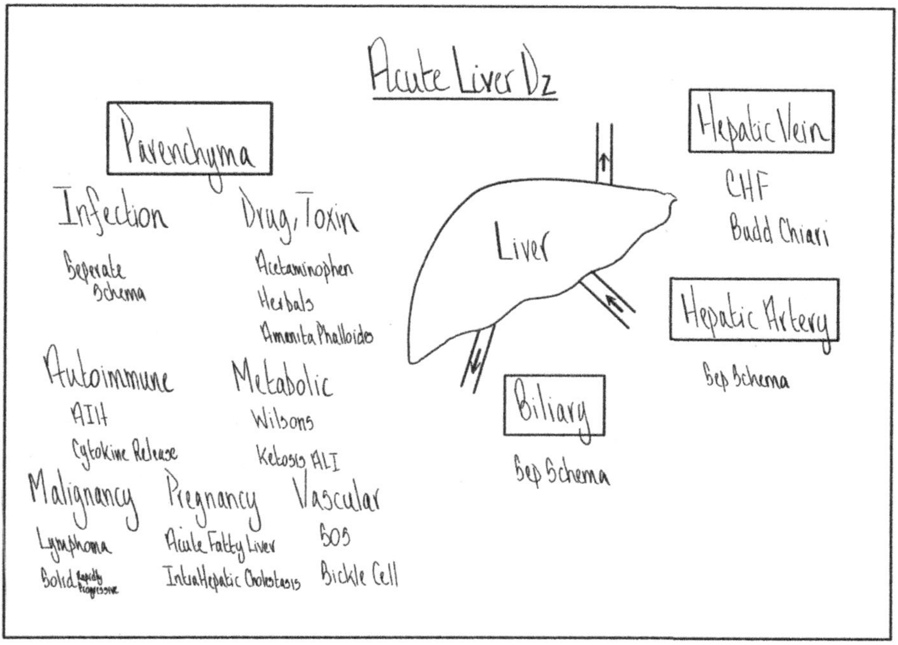

This figure organizes acute liver disease by anatomic compartment: parenchyma, arterial inflow, venous outflow, and biliary system. The central diagnostic task is to localize the site of injury before identifying the cause.

Parenchymal disease reflects direct hepatocyte injury or infiltration. Viral hepatitis remains the most common cause. Drug- and toxin-induced injury is a critical consideration, particularly acetaminophen toxicity, which can lead to rapid liver failure, as well as herbal supplements and other hepatotoxins. Autoimmune hepatitis, metabolic disorders such as Wilson disease, and systemic inflammatory states may also produce acute hepatocellular injury. Infiltrative processes, including malignancy, can impair hepatic function through replacement or disruption of normal architecture.

Arterial causes reflect impaired hepatic perfusion. Hypotension, shock, or low-flow states lead to ischemic injury with marked aminotransferase elevation. These processes are often transient, with rapid improvement following restoration of perfusion.

Venous outflow obstruction results in hepatic congestion. Congestive heart failure produces passive congestion, while Budd–Chiari syndrome reflects hepatic vein thrombosis or obstruction. Both lead to hepatomegaly, impaired drainage, and progressive liver dysfunction.

Biliary causes arise from obstruction and cholestasis. Gallstones are the most common etiology, while malignancy or strictures may produce similar patterns. These processes often present with jaundice and require imaging to identify the site of obstruction and guide intervention.

This framework emphasizes localization before labeling. Identifying whether injury arises from hepatocytes, inflow, outflow, or biliary obstruction clarifies mechanism and directs evaluation and management.

Figure 14.2

Ischemic hepatitis: pattern + physiology

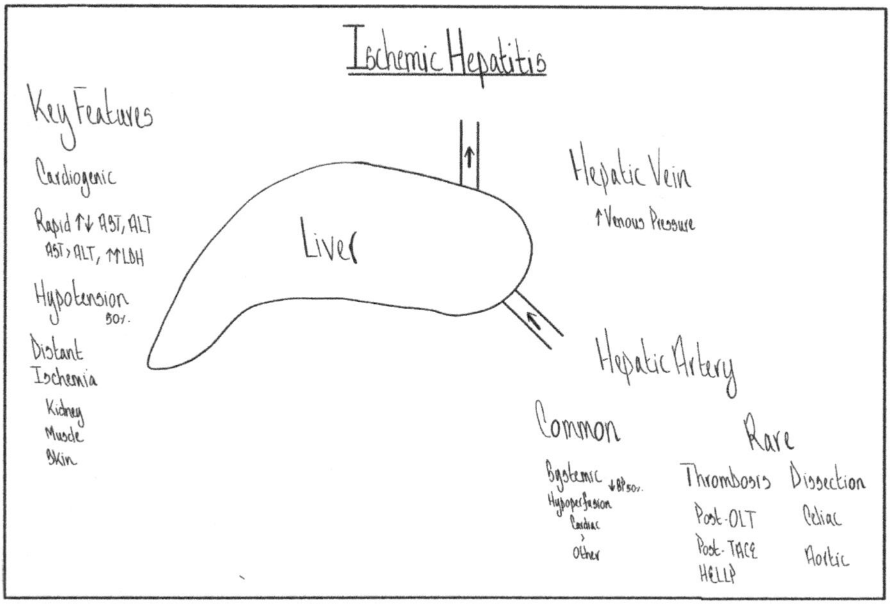

This figure organizes ischemic hepatitis by vascular mechanism, distinguishing impaired arterial inflow from impaired venous outflow. The central diagnostic task is to identify a preceding low-flow state.

Arterial causes are most common and typically reflect systemic hypoperfusion. Cardiac conditions—such as arrhythmias, myocardial infarction, or other low-output states—lead to reduced hepatic oxygen delivery and hepatocellular injury. This produces a characteristic pattern of marked aminotransferase elevation with disproportionate LDH rise, followed by rapid improvement once perfusion is restored. The tempo of recovery is a key distinguishing feature.

Less commonly, ischemic hepatitis results from primary arterial compromise. Hepatic artery thrombosis, most often seen after liver transplantation or vascular procedures, can cause abrupt ischemia. Other rare vascular insults, including arterial dissection or pregnancy-related microvascular disease, may similarly impair hepatic inflow.

Venous causes reflect impaired outflow and hepatic congestion. Congestive heart failure leads to passive congestion and reduced effective perfusion, while Budd–Chiari syndrome involves hepatic vein thrombosis or obstruction. Despite differing mechanisms, both produce a similar biochemical pattern of acute liver injury.

Ischemic hepatitis often occurs in the context of systemic hypoperfusion. Concurrent organ injury—such as acute kidney injury or muscle injury—supports a global low-flow state. Importantly, hypotension may be transient or undocumented, and its absence at presentation does not exclude the diagnosis.

This framework emphasizes reconstruction of the hemodynamic event. Identifying whether injury arises from impaired inflow or outflow—and recognizing the systemic context—guides diagnosis and management.

Figure 15.1
Hypotension: Arterial Pressure and Venous Pressure

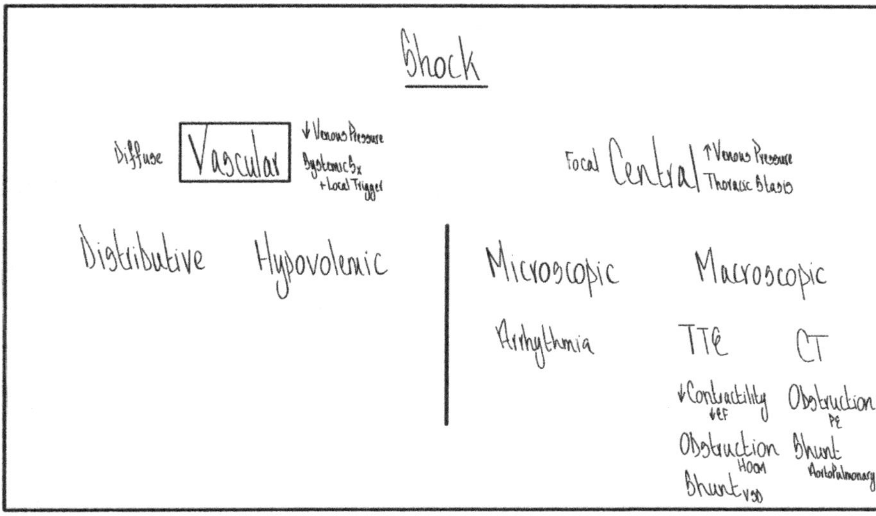

This figure organizes shock using venous pressure as the initial diagnostic pivot. The central task is to determine whether venous pressure is low or elevated at the bedside.

Low venous pressure reflects inadequate effective circulating volume and frames shock as a diffuse vascular problem. Findings such as flat neck veins and tachycardia suggest reduced preload. Cool extremities point toward hypovolemia, reflecting compensatory vasoconstriction, whereas distributive shock—most commonly sepsis—typically presents with warm extremities due to pathologic vasodilation. In this branch, evaluation focuses on identifying sources of fluid loss or systemic infection.

Elevated venous pressure indicates impaired forward flow despite adequate or increased filling, reflecting a central circulatory problem. This may result from pump failure or obstruction to cardiac inflow or outflow. Rhythm disturbances and loss of atrioventricular synchrony can reduce cardiac output at a microscopic level. More commonly, macroscopic processes dominate, including cardiogenic shock from impaired contractility, or obstructive shock from conditions such as pulmonary embolism, cardiac tamponade, or tension pneumothorax. These processes lead to congestion upstream and hypotension downstream.

Bedside imaging refines this distinction. Echocardiography can identify reduced ejection fraction, outflow obstruction, or chamber dilation, while additional imaging may reveal structural or obstructive pathology. However, the initial classification is clinical: low versus high venous pressure.

This framework emphasizes a central principle: assess venous pressure to rapidly localize the mechanism of shock. Distinguishing diffuse volume loss from impaired forward flow guides immediate management and prioritizes further evaluation.

Figure 15.2
Atrioventricular Block: Integrity of Conduction

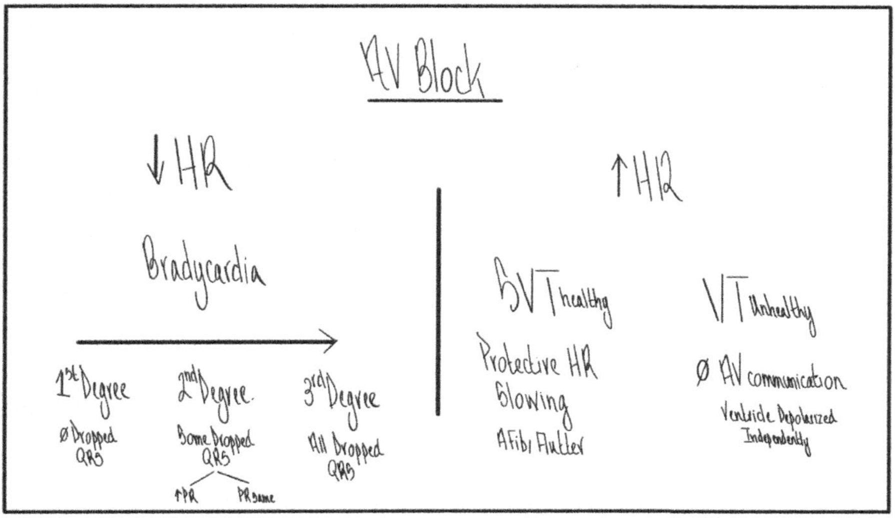

Atrioventricular (AV) block represents impaired conduction between the atria and ventricles and is best organized by its effect on conduction and degree of block. The central diagnostic task is to determine the level and severity of conduction failure.

Bradycardia due to AV block is most common and reflects progressive impairment of conduction. First-degree AV block is defined by a prolonged PR interval with preserved conduction of all atrial impulses. Second-degree AV block introduces intermittent failure of conduction, resulting in dropped beats. Third-degree (complete) AV block represents total dissociation between atrial and ventricular activity, with ventricular escape rhythms maintaining cardiac output.

Second-degree AV block is further divided into two patterns. Mobitz type I (Wenckebach) is characterized by progressive PR prolongation before a dropped beat and typically localizes to the AV node, often reflecting a reversible or benign process. Mobitz type II presents with sudden dropped beats without prior PR prolongation and usually reflects disease below the AV node; it carries a higher risk of progression to complete heart block and often requires urgent intervention. In 2:1 AV block, distinguishing these patterns relies on rhythm regularity and clinical context.

Common causes of AV block include medications that impair conduction (such as beta-blockers, calcium channel blockers, and digoxin), electrolyte disturbances (particularly hyperkalemia), and myocardial ischemia involving the conduction system. Degenerative and infiltrative processes may also contribute.

In tachyarrhythmias, AV dissociation can also occur. Ventricular tachycardia produces independent ventricular activation, with occasional capture or fusion beats supporting the diagnosis. In supraventricular tachycardias, the AV node may act as a protective filter, limiting conduction of rapid atrial impulses to the ventricles.

This framework emphasizes pattern recognition. Identifying the degree of block and its conduction pattern localizes the defect and guides urgency of management.

Figure 16.1
Anasarca

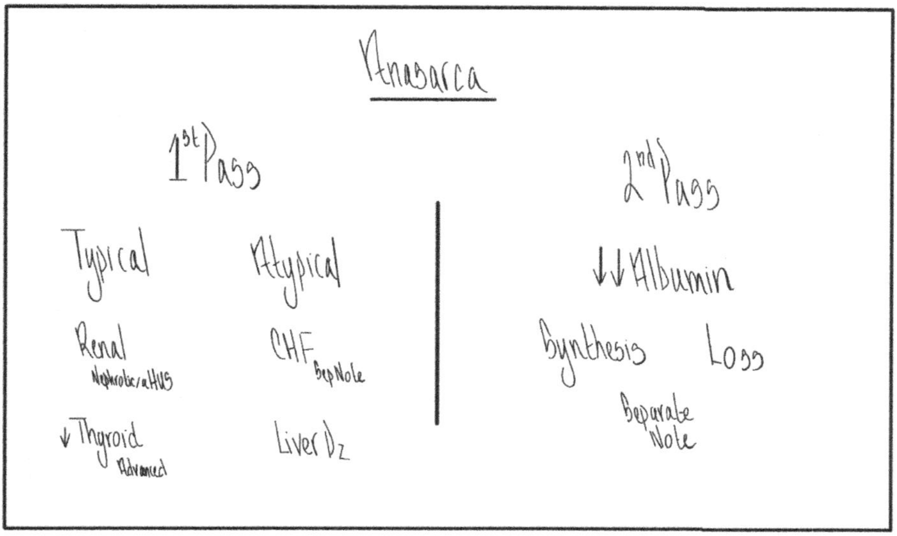

This figure organizes anasarca as generalized edema involving multiple compartments, distinguishing it from isolated dependent swelling. The central diagnostic task is to identify common causes before evaluating underlying mechanisms.

The first pass prioritizes typical etiologies. Renal disease—particularly nephrotic syndrome—is a leading cause, along with endocrine disorders such as hypothyroidism. In all patients, evaluation should include assessment of proteinuria and measurement of thyroid-stimulating hormone. Cardiac and hepatic disease may also contribute: while heart failure and liver disease often produce dependent edema, severe or advanced states can result in generalized swelling. Medications, including nonsteroidal anti-inflammatory drugs, calcium channel blockers, thiazolidinediones, and corticosteroids, may also promote fluid retention.

If initial evaluation is unrevealing, a second pass focuses on mechanism, particularly hypoalbuminemia. Reduced oncotic pressure may result from decreased synthesis, as seen in advanced liver disease or systemic inflammation, or from increased loss through the kidneys, gastrointestinal tract, or vascular leak states.

This framework emphasizes a stepwise approach: first identify common causes, then define the underlying mechanism. Recognizing whether anasarca reflects organ dysfunction or altered oncotic balance guides further evaluation and management.

Figure 16.2
Approaching Hypoalbuminemia

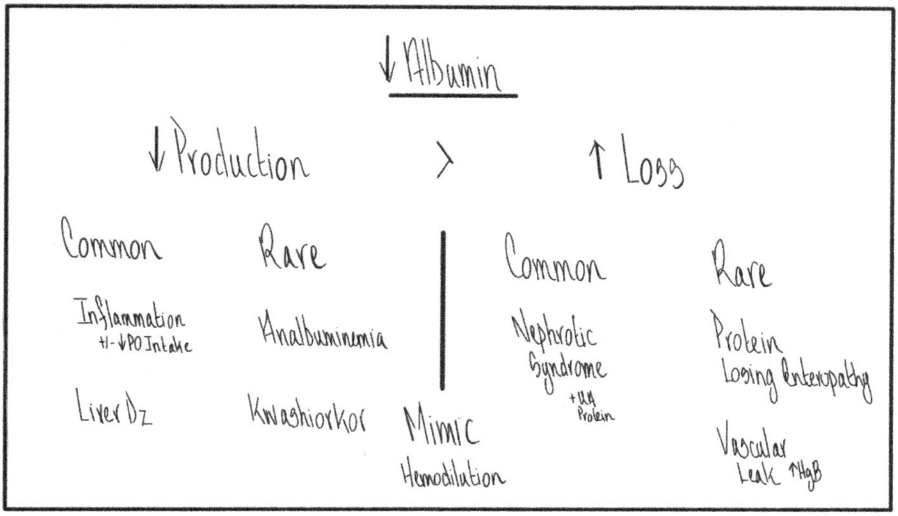

This figure organizes hypoalbuminemia using a stepwise approach: assess severity, then determine mechanism. The central diagnostic task is to distinguish decreased production from increased loss.

Mild hypoalbuminemia (approximately 3–3.5 g/dL) is common and most often reflects chronic inflammation or malnutrition. In the absence of concerning features, extensive evaluation is typically unnecessary. More significant hypoalbuminemia (less than 3 g/dL), particularly when accompanied by edema or other abnormalities, warrants further investigation.

Decreased production is the most common mechanism. Systemic inflammation shifts hepatic synthesis toward acute-phase proteins and away from albumin, often in the setting of chronic illness or infection. Advanced liver disease also reduces albumin synthesis. Less common causes include severe protein malnutrition and rare genetic disorders affecting albumin production.

Increased loss is less common but clinically important. Renal loss, as seen in nephrotic syndrome, is the classic cause and should be suspected when hypoalbuminemia is accompanied by edema; urinalysis is essential in this setting. Gastrointestinal loss occurs in protein-losing enteropathy due to mucosal or lymphatic disease. Vascular leak states represent a third mechanism, in which albumin escapes into the interstitial space, often in the context of systemic illness.

Apparent hypoalbuminemia may also result from hemodilution. Increased plasma volume, as seen in pregnancy or fluid overload, can lower measured albumin without true loss.

This framework emphasizes mechanism after severity. Identifying whether hypoalbuminemia reflects reduced synthesis, increased loss, or dilution guides evaluation and management.

Figure 17.1
Disseminated Lymphadenopathy

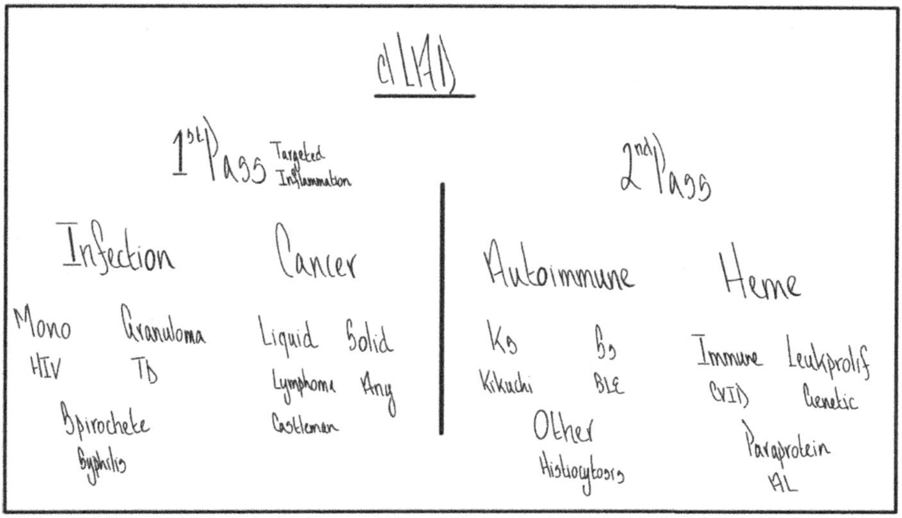

This figure organizes disseminated lymphadenopathy using a two-pass framework. The central diagnostic task is to distinguish processes driven by an identifiable stimulus from those arising from dysregulated host biology.

The first pass prioritizes stimulus-driven etiologies, particularly infection and malignancy. Infectious causes commonly produce generalized immune activation. Viral infections, especially mononucleosis-like syndromes due to Epstein–Barr virus, cytomegalovirus, or human immunodeficiency virus, are frequent. Granulomatous infections, such as tuberculosis or endemic fungi, may present similarly. Spirochetal infections, including syphilis, are additional considerations. Malignancy is a key cause of diffuse lymphadenopathy and includes both lymphoid processes (such as lymphoma and Castleman disease) and metastatic solid tumors.

The second pass considers processes arising from dysregulated or systemic immune biology. Systemic autoimmune diseases, including systemic lupus erythematosus and Sjögren syndrome, can cause persistent lymphadenopathy through chronic immune activation. Granulomatous diseases such as sarcoidosis and self-limited conditions like Kikuchi disease may present with similar findings. Disorders of immune regulation, including hemophagocytic syndromes or immunodeficiency states, can also produce widespread nodal enlargement.

Mimics should also be considered. Dermatopathic lymphadenopathy represents a benign, reactive process associated with chronic skin disease and may resemble systemic pathology.

This framework emphasizes a stepwise approach: first identify processes driven by infection or malignancy, then consider systemic or dysregulated immune conditions. When lymphadenopathy involves multiple regions, particularly deep nodal stations without a clear explanation, malignancy—both lymphoid and metastatic—should remain a central consideration and prompt further evaluation.

Figure 17.2
Lymphadenopathy Diagnosable Without Biopsy

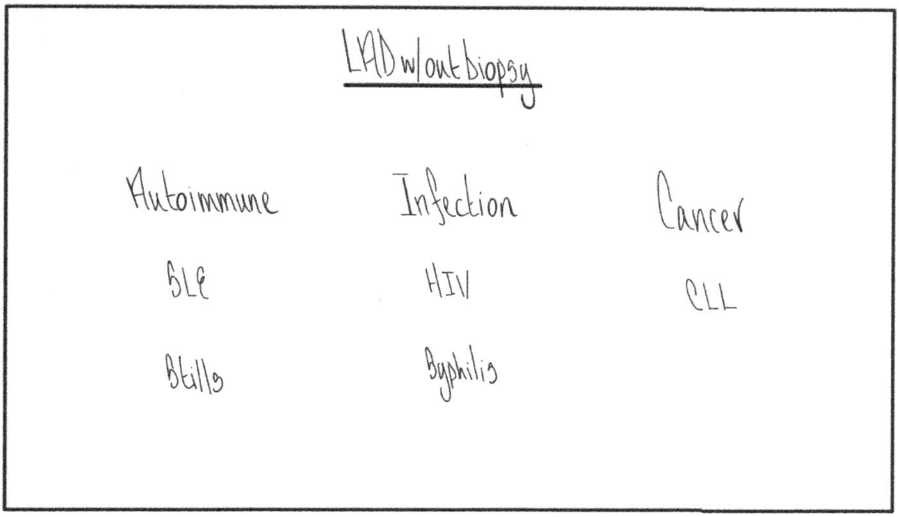

This figure highlights conditions in which lymphadenopathy can be diagnosed through blood testing, reducing the need for immediate tissue biopsy. The central task is to identify systemic processes detectable through noninvasive evaluation.

Infectious causes are among the most readily identified. Human immunodeficiency virus and syphilis commonly produce diffuse lymphadenopathy and can be diagnosed through serologic testing.

Hematologic malignancies may also be detected through peripheral blood evaluation. Chronic lymphocytic leukemia often presents with lymphadenopathy and characteristic lymphocytosis, allowing diagnosis without lymph node biopsy in many cases.

Autoimmune conditions represent another category. Diseases such as systemic lupus erythematosus can produce generalized lymphadenopathy and are often identified through serologic markers.

This framework emphasizes a practical principle: when lymphadenopathy reflects a systemic process, blood testing may establish the diagnosis before invasive evaluation is pursued.

Figure 18.1
Differential Diagnosis of Hypothermia

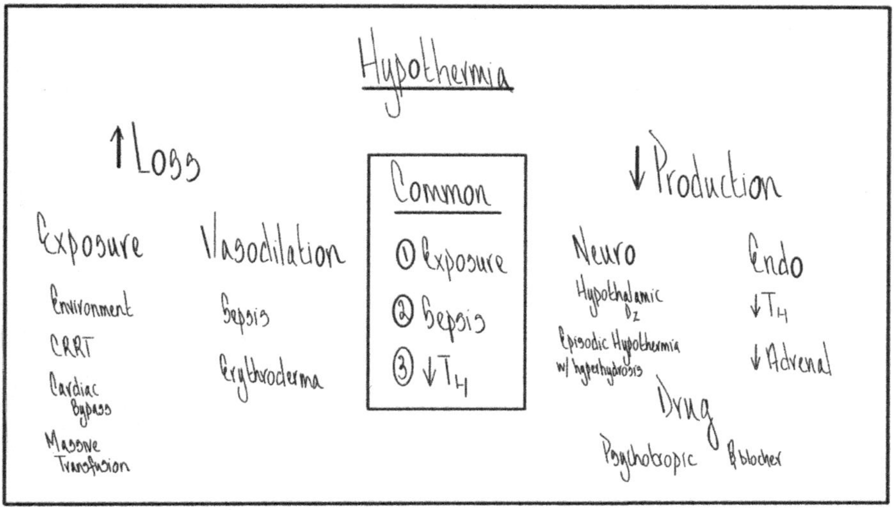

This figure organizes severe hypothermia by mechanism, distinguishing increased heat loss from decreased heat production. The central diagnostic task is to identify which process predominates.

Increased heat loss most commonly results from environmental exposure, including cold environments, immersion, or inadequate protection, and remains the most frequent cause overall. Medical settings can also contribute, particularly during extracorporeal therapies or massive transfusion. Peripheral vasodilation further amplifies heat loss by directing blood flow to the skin; this is commonly seen in sepsis and inflammatory skin disorders such as erythroderma.

Decreased heat production reflects impaired thermoregulation or reduced metabolic activity. Endocrine disorders—most notably hypothyroidism—are among the most common causes in this category and reduce basal heat generation. Neurologic causes, particularly hypothalamic dysfunction, disrupt central temperature control. Hypercapnia also contributes by depressing central respiratory drive and metabolic activity, often coexisting with hypoventilation syndromes. Medications, especially psychotropic agents and beta-blockers, can further blunt physiologic and behavioral responses to cold.

This framework emphasizes mechanism over setting. Severe hypothermia arises from either excessive heat loss or impaired heat generation, and distinguishing between these processes—while recognizing common contributors such as environmental exposure, sepsis, and hypothyroidism—guides evaluation and management.

Figure 18.2
Causes of Hypoventilation

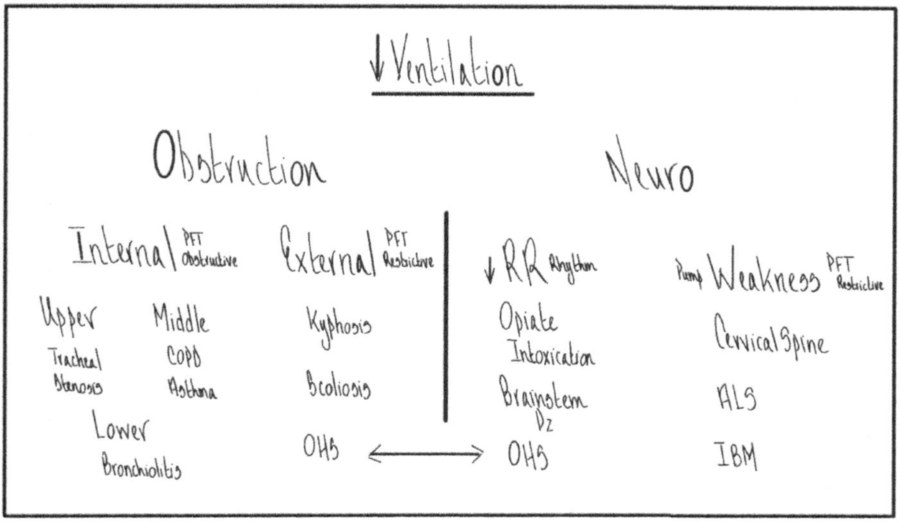

This figure organizes hypoventilation by mechanism, distinguishing obstructive from neurogenic causes. The central diagnostic task is to identify why alveolar ventilation is reduced, leading to hypercapnia.

Obstructive causes reflect impaired airflow. Internal airway obstruction produces an obstructive pattern on pulmonary function testing and may occur at any level: upper airway narrowing (e.g., tracheal stenosis), large airway disease such as asthma or chronic obstructive pulmonary disease, or small airway inflammation. External restriction limits chest wall expansion and reduces ventilation, producing a restrictive pattern. Common causes include chest wall deformities and obesity hypoventilation, where excess body mass impairs respiratory mechanics.

Neurogenic causes reflect impaired control or execution of breathing. Disorders of respiratory rhythm reduce central drive, as seen with opioid intoxication or brainstem disease. Disorders of the respiratory pump involve muscle weakness, limiting effective ventilation despite preserved drive. These include neuromuscular conditions affecting the diaphragm and accessory muscles.

This framework emphasizes mechanism over location. Whether due to airflow limitation or impaired respiratory drive or effort, all forms of hypoventilation result in reduced ventilation and carbon dioxide retention, guiding evaluation and management.

Figure 19.1
PEA Arrest

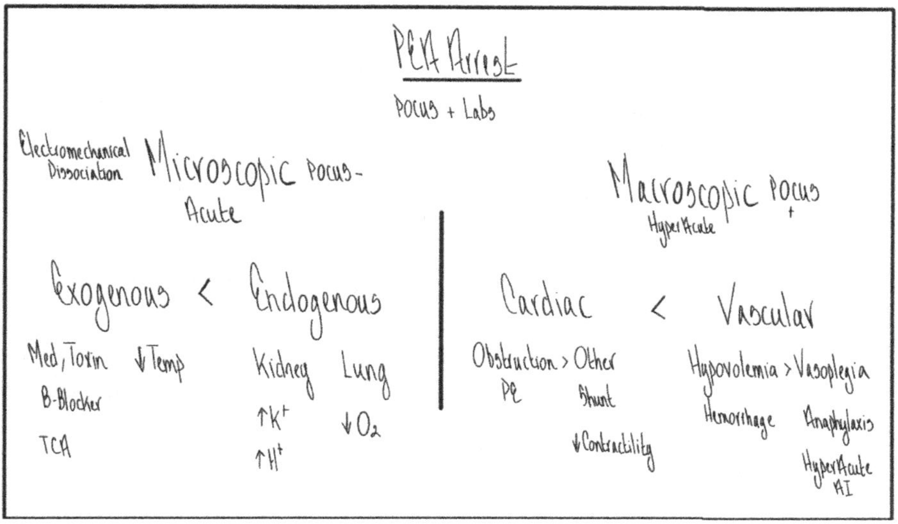

This figure organizes pulseless electrical activity (PEA) by mechanism, distinguishing microscopic (POCUS-negative) from macroscopic (POCUS-positive) causes. The central diagnostic task is to identify why organized electrical activity fails to generate effective perfusion.

Microscopic causes are POCUS-negative and reflect electrical–mechanical dissociation at the cellular level. Cardiac motion may be present, but contractility is insufficient to produce a pulse. These processes are typically acute in tempo and are further divided into exogenous and endogenous drivers. Exogenous causes include toxins and medications—such as beta-blockers and tricyclic antidepressants—as well as hypothermia, all of which impair cellular energy utilization or myocardial responsiveness. Endogenous causes arise from internal physiologic failure, most commonly renal and pulmonary derangements, including hyperkalemia, acidemia, and hypoxemia. In this branch, laboratory evaluation is essential to rapidly identify and reverse metabolic abnormalities.

Macroscopic causes are POCUS-positive and reflect structural or hemodynamic failure of circulation. These processes are typically hyperacute in tempo, leading to abrupt loss of effective cardiac output. Cardiac causes include obstructive processes such as pulmonary embolism and cardiac tamponade, as well as severe reductions in contractility or pathologic shunts. Vascular causes include hypovolemia—most often due to hemorrhage—and distributive states such as vasoplegia or anaphylaxis. In this branch, POCUS is essential for rapid localization and targeted intervention.

This framework emphasizes a central principle: use ultrasound and tempo to distinguish cellular failure from structural collapse. Identifying whether PEA is POCUS-negative (acute, microscopic) or POCUS-positive (hyperacute, macroscopic) guides immediate resuscitation and prioritizes reversible causes.

Figure 19.2
Cath-Negative ACS

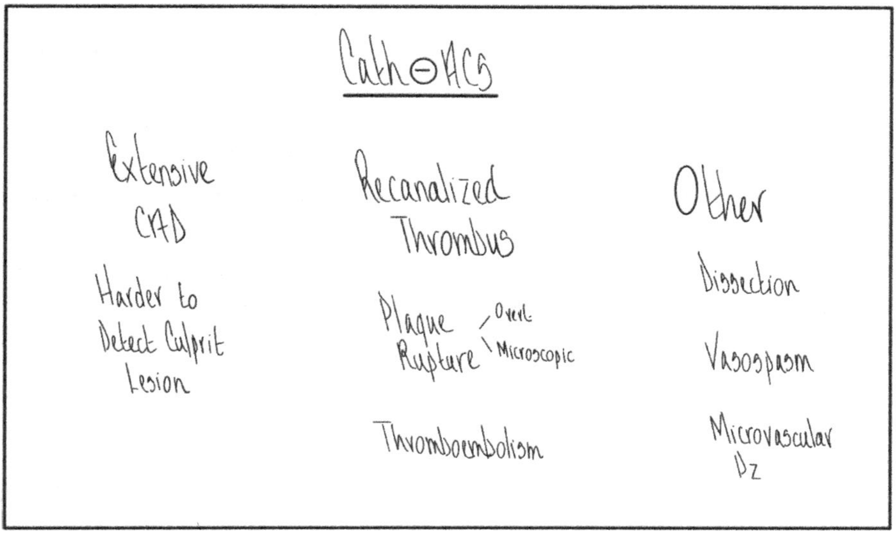

This figure organizes catheterization-negative acute coronary syndrome as ischemia without an identifiable culprit lesion on angiography. The central diagnostic task is to determine the mechanism of transient or non-obstructive coronary flow impairment.

One major mechanism is transient occlusion. A thrombus may form and then recanalize before angiography, leaving minimal or no visible abnormality. Similarly, embolic material from a proximal source may temporarily obstruct coronary flow and then resolve or migrate distally.

Intrinsic coronary processes may also be missed on routine angiography. Coronary vasospasm produces abrupt, reversible constriction without fixed obstruction. Subtle dissection or in-situ thrombosis can impair flow but may not be apparent if luminal narrowing is minimal or transient.

Microvascular dysfunction represents another important category. Ischemia may arise from impaired flow at the level of small vessels or from microembolization, leading to symptoms and biomarker elevation despite normal epicardial arteries.

Finally, diffuse coronary disease may obscure a clear culprit lesion, with multiple areas of abnormality preventing identification of a single responsible site.

This framework encourages clinicians to consider a broad range of physiological and anatomical contributors when angiography does not reveal a clear culprit lesion. By focusing on transient occlusion, vasomotor disturbances, microvascular dysfunction, and diffuse coronary disease, the approach integrates both mechanism and anatomy to guide further evaluation and management.

Figure 20.1
Acute Hypertension with Neurologic Symptoms

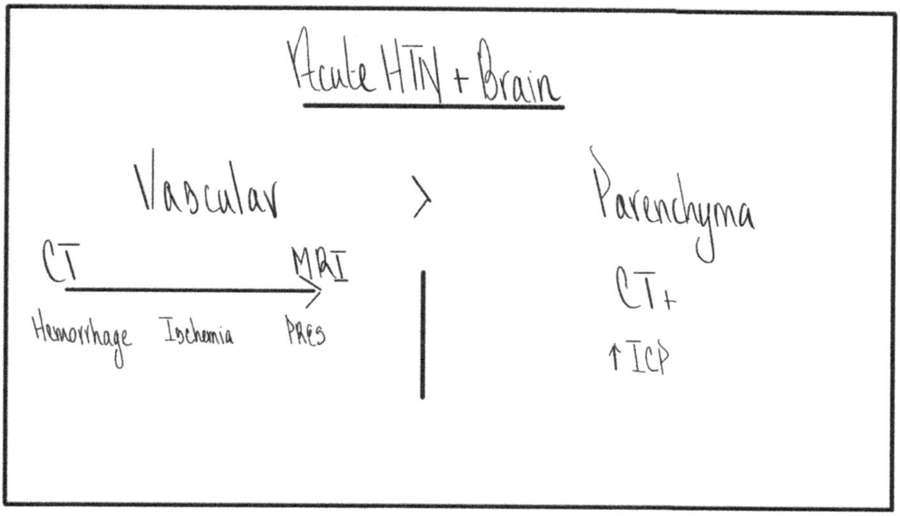

This figure organizes acute hypertension with neurologic symptoms by mechanism, distinguishing vascular events from parenchymal processes. The central diagnostic task is to determine whether hypertension is the cause of neurologic injury or a response to it.

Vascular causes reflect primary disturbances of cerebral blood flow. Intracranial hemorrhage, including hypertensive hemorrhage and subarachnoid hemorrhage, presents with abrupt neurologic symptoms and elevated blood pressure. Acute ischemic stroke may also be associated with hypertension, which often represents a compensatory response to maintain cerebral perfusion. Posterior reversible encephalopathy syndrome arises from failure of autoregulation in the setting of severe hypertension, leading to headache, visual disturbance, confusion, or seizures.

Parenchymal processes reflect structural or inflammatory disease within the brain. Mass lesions, cerebral edema, infection, or inflammatory conditions increase intracranial pressure and disrupt normal function. In these cases, hypertension is often secondary, driven by sympathetic activation in response to rising intracranial pressure.

This framework emphasizes a key diagnostic distinction: hypertension may be the driver of neurologic injury or a physiologic response to intracranial disease. Early imaging is essential to differentiate these mechanisms and guide management.

Figure 20.2
Mechanisms of Hyponatremia

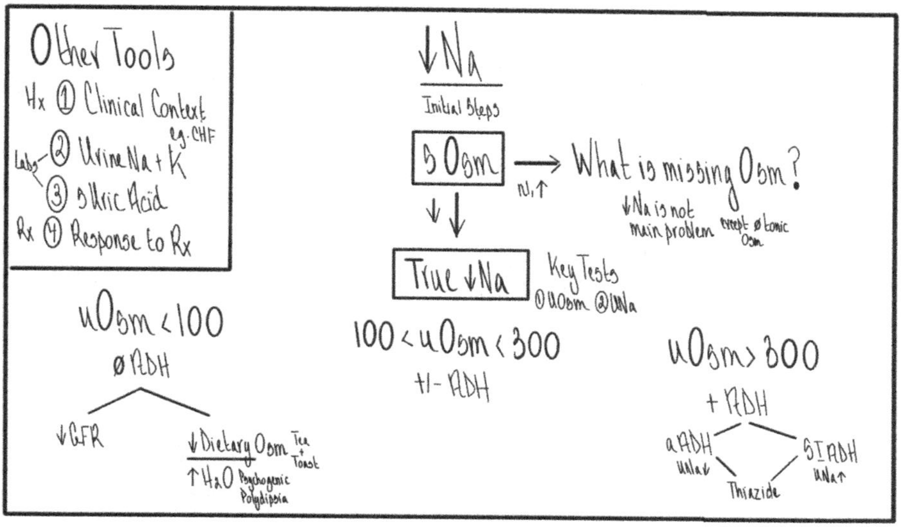

This figure organizes hyponatremia using a stepwise physiologic approach. The central diagnostic task is to determine whether low sodium reflects true hypotonicity and, if so, why water excretion is impaired.

Initial evaluation begins with clinical context and severity. Mild hyponatremia typically requires only a focused evaluation. More significant or unexplained cases warrant confirmation of hypotonic hyponatremia with measurement of serum osmolality. Normal or elevated osmolality suggests alternative processes, including hyperglycemia or laboratory artifact from hyperproteinemia or hyperlipidemia.

Once hypotonic hyponatremia is confirmed, urine osmolality defines the next branch point. A low urine osmolality indicates suppression of antidiuretic hormone and appropriate free water excretion, most often due to excess water intake or low solute states. A higher urine osmolality indicates active antidiuretic hormone and impaired water clearance.

In this setting, urine sodium and clinical context determine whether antidiuretic hormone activity is appropriate or inappropriate. Low urine sodium suggests volume depletion or reduced effective circulating volume, as seen in hypovolemia, heart failure, or cirrhosis. Higher urine sodium with ongoing natriuresis suggests inappropriate hormone activity, as in the syndrome of inappropriate antidiuretic hormone secretion. Certain conditions, including diuretic use or intrinsic renal injury, may blur this distinction.

Response to therapy provides additional clarity. Improvement with isotonic fluids supports hypovolemia-mediated hormone release, whereas lack of response or worsening hyponatremia suggests inappropriate antidiuretic hormone activity.

This framework emphasizes physiology over labeling. Determining whether antidiuretic hormone is suppressed, appropriately activated, or misfiring localizes the mechanism and guides management.

Figure 21.1
Orthostasis Clues

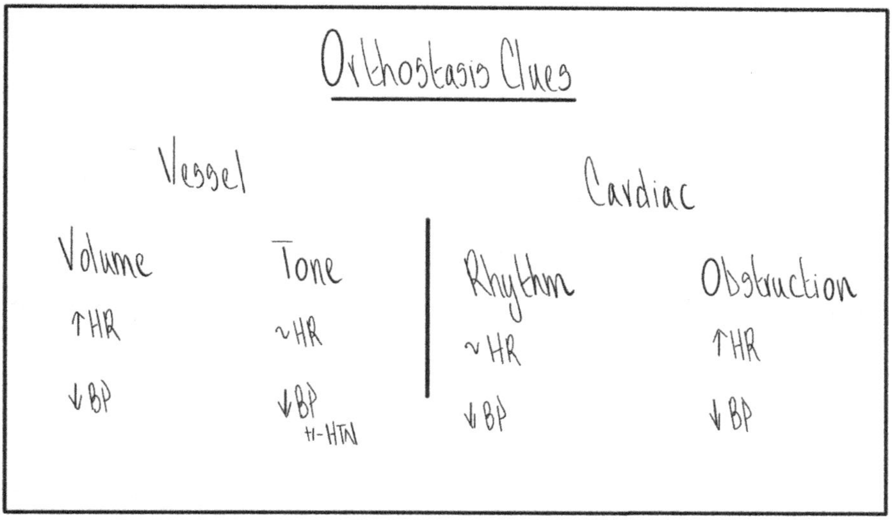

This figure organizes orthostatic hypotension by mechanism, using the heart rate response to distinguish impaired volume, vascular tone, or cardiac output. The central diagnostic task is to determine whether the compensatory response to standing is intact.

Normally, standing shifts blood to the lower extremities, reducing venous return. Baroreceptor-mediated sympathetic activation increases heart rate and vascular tone to maintain perfusion. Orthostatic hypotension occurs when this response is inadequate.

Vessel-related causes are most common. Hypovolemia leads to reduced preload and a compensatory rise in heart rate. In contrast, autonomic dysfunction results in loss of vascular tone with an absent or blunted heart rate response. This may occur with medications or conditions such as diabetes affecting autonomic pathways, and may be accompanied by baseline or supine hypertension.

Cardiac causes reflect impaired ability to augment output. Rhythm disturbances, including bradyarrhythmias or conduction disease, prevent appropriate heart rate increase. Structural conditions that limit forward flow, such as fixed outflow obstruction or restrictive physiology, may produce a similar pattern.

Obstructive processes impair venous return or cardiac filling. In these cases, heart rate is typically elevated, but blood pressure remains low due to mechanical limitation of flow.

This framework emphasizes pattern recognition at the bedside. Interpreting the relationship between heart rate and blood pressure during standing localizes the mechanism and guides further evaluation.

Figure 21.2

Subacute Peritoneal Disease

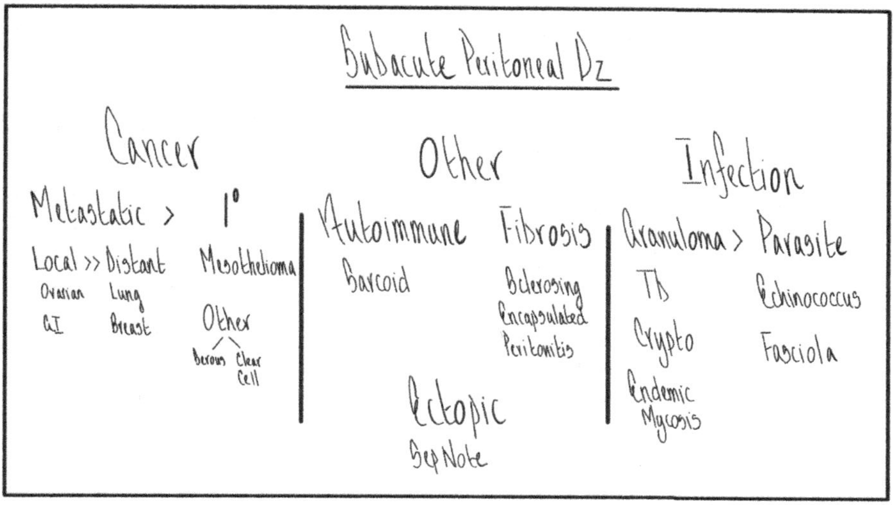

This figure organizes subacute peritoneal disease into three major categories: malignant, infectious, and other inflammatory or infiltrative processes. The central diagnostic task is to distinguish among these etiologies using clinical context, imaging, and peritoneal fluid analysis.

Malignancy is the most common cause. Peritoneal involvement typically reflects metastatic disease, most often from ovarian or gastrointestinal primaries. Peritoneal carcinomatosis may present with ascites, peritoneal thickening, and omental caking. Primary peritoneal malignancies are less common but should be considered when imaging resembles ovarian cancer without a clear ovarian source.

Infectious causes are most often granulomatous. Tuberculous peritonitis and endemic fungal infections can closely mimic malignancy, producing similar imaging findings and subacute symptoms. These diagnoses are particularly relevant in immunocompromised patients or endemic regions. Parasitic infections are less common but may present with cystic or inflammatory peritoneal involvement.

Other causes include autoimmune and fibrosing disorders. Conditions such as sarcoidosis may produce granulomatous inflammation, while fibrosing processes can lead to peritoneal thickening and bowel encasement. Ectopic processes, including endometriosis, may also involve the peritoneum and present with chronic or subacute symptoms.

Because clinical and imaging features often overlap, definitive diagnosis frequently requires integration of fluid analysis and tissue biopsy.

This framework emphasizes categorization before confirmation. Distinguishing malignant, infectious, and inflammatory causes guides diagnostic testing and directs management.

Made in the USA
Las Vegas, NV
01 November 2026

57090823R00164